Psychotherapeutic Competencies

This book provides a clear and concise description of the multifaceted notion of psychotherapeutic competencies, building on years of research and training and informed by a systemic approach.

Psychotherapeutic Competencies clearly describes methodological principles to guide both trainees and experienced therapists through the definition of four levels of systemic competencies and illustrates each principle with compelling clinical case material. The book emphasises the need for therapists to develop relational skills, which allow for the consolidation of a trusting relationship in which change can take place, as well as acquiring a set of methods and techniques. *Psychotherapeutic Competencies* encourages therapists of all levels of experience and therapeutic backgrounds to develop epistemological competency and to deepen their awareness of the extended contexts in which they operate and of the possible effects of their practice at a social and cultural level.

This book will be essential reading for psychotherapists of all therapeutic backgrounds, in practice and in training, who wish to enhance their understanding of competency, context, and clinical skill. It will also be a key text for systemic and relational psychotherapists, trainers, trainees, clinical supervisors, and researchers.

Laura Fruggeri is a psychologist and psychotherapist and a former professor of psychology of family relationship at the University of Parma. Currently, she is the director of the Bologna Centre of Family Therapy and has been extensively teaching in the UK, Europe, and North and South America for more than 3 decades. She is the author of more than 100 publications in Italian, English, French, Spanish, Danish, and German.

Francesca Balestra, PhD, is a psychologist and psychotherapist. She is a family therapist, a researcher, and a trainer at the Bologna Centre of Family Therapy. Her research interests are focused on communicative and interactive processes between therapist and client in psychotherapeutic sessions.

Elena Venturelli, PhD, is a psychologist and psychotherapist, adjunct professor of psychology of family relationships at the University of Parma, and a researcher and trainer at the Bologna Centre of Family Therapy. Her main research interests are relationships in the family, with particular attention to the analysis of interactions through observational methodologies (TIAP).

The Systemic Thinking and Practice Series
Series Editors: Charlotte Burck and Gwyn Daniel

This influential series was co-founded in 1989 by series editors David Campbell and Ros Draper to promote innovative applications of systemic theory to psychotherapy, teaching, supervision and organisational consultation. In 2011, Charlotte Burck and Gwyn Daniel became series editors and aim to present new theoretical developments and pioneering practice, to make links with other theoretical approaches, and to promote the relevance of systemic theory to contemporary social and psychological questions.

Recent titles in the series include:

Surviving and Thriving in Care and Beyond: Personal and Professional Perspectives
Edited by Sara Barratt and Wendy Lobatto

Emotions and the Therapist: A Systemic-Dialogical Approach
By Paolo Bertrando

Creative Positions in Adult Mental Health: Outside In-Inside Out
Edited by Sue McNab and Karen Partridge

Ethical and Aesthetic Explorations of Systemic Practice: New Critical Reflections
Pietro Barbetta, Maria Esther Cavagnis, Inga-Britt Krause, and Umberta Telfener

Working Systemically with Refugee Couples and Families: Exploring Trauma, Resilience and Culture
Shadi Shahnavaz

Psychotherapeutic Competencies: Techniques, Relationships, and Epistemology in Systemic Practice
Laura Fruggeri, Francesca Balestra, and Elena Venturelli

"This excellent book is a guide to becoming competent in using systemic therapy to help individuals, couples, and families. It integrates key themes from the fields of psychotherapy and research. Complex ideas and practices are illustrated with case examples. This book is a gem, clearly written, insightful, and a 'must read' for students, trainers, and experienced couple and family therapists."

Professor Alan Carr, *University College Dublin*

"Building on the senior author's outstanding scholarship, *Psychotherapeutic Competencies* illuminates the conceptual cores of *avant garde* systemic practices, to then anchoring them with vivid excerpts of clinical practice. A brilliant, important book."

Carlos E. Sluzki, *MD George Washington University*

"*Psychotherapeutic Competencies* is an appetizing addition to the menu of psychotherapy, appealing to many palates. Traditional dishes from systemic practice: hypothesizing, curiosity, and questions are refreshed and enhanced by contemporary flavours of therapeutic relationships and spiced by research and evidence."

John Burnham, *Birmingham Women's and Children's Hospital*

Psychotherapeutic Competencies

Techniques, Relationships, and
Epistemology in Systemic Practice

**Laura Fruggeri,
Francesca Balestra, and
Elena Venturelli**

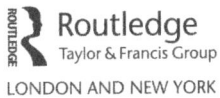
LONDON AND NEW YORK

Cover image: From Getty

First published 2023
by Routledge
4 Park Square, Milton Park, Abingdon, Oxon OX14 4RN

and by Routledge
605 Third Avenue, New York, NY 10158

Routledge is an imprint of the Taylor & Francis Group, an informa business

British Library Cataloguing-in-Publication Data
A catalogue record for this book is available from the British Library

Library of Congress Cataloging-in-Publication Data
Names: Fruggeri, Laura, author. | Balestra, Francesca, author. | Venturelli,
Elena, author.
Title: Psychotherapeutic competencies : techniques, relationships, and
epistemology in systemic practice / Laura Fruggeri, Francesca Balestra, and
Elena Venturelli.
Description: First edition. | Abingdon, Oxon ; New York, NY : Routledge,
2023. | Series: The systemic thinking and practice series | Includes
bibliographical references and index.
Identifiers: LCCN 2022025567 (print) | LCCN 2022025568 (ebook) |
ISBN 9781032235288 (hbk) | ISBN 9781032235264 (pbk) | ISBN
9781003278092 (ebk)
Subjects: LCSH: Psychotherapist and patient. |
Psychotherapists--Training of.
Classification: LCC RC480.8 .F78 2023 (print) | LCC RC480.8 (ebook) |
DDC 616.89/14--dc23/eng/20220720
LC record available at https://lccn.loc.gov/2022025567
LC ebook record available at https://lccn.loc.gov/2022025568

ISBN: 978-1-032-23528-8 (hbk)
ISBN: 978-1-032-23526-4 (pbk)
ISBN: 978-1-003-27809-2 (ebk)

DOI: 10.4324/9781003278092

Typeset in Bembo
by MPS Limited, Dehradun

Contents

Series Editors' Foreword by Charlotte Burck and Gwyn Daniel   ix
Foreword by Imelda McCarthy   xi
Preface   xvii
Acknowledgements   xix

Introduction: specific and common factors of
psychotherapy   1

PART I
**Technical competency in systemic practice: the
dialogical construction of a shared symbolic space**   17

1   From diagnosis to care   19

2   Technical support for dialogical competency   36

PART II
**Relational competency: promoting and analyzing
intersubjectivity**   55

3   The therapeutic alliance   57

4   The construction of transformative interactive contexts   75

PART III
**Epistemological competency: the ability to change
point of view**   95

5   Reflexivity: becoming aware of one's own premises   97

6   Complex thinking: the exploration of different perspectives   113

7   Curiosity and decentring: distinguishing reasons from
    solutions   127

PART IV
Acknowledging the context: the social dimension of
psychotherapy   139

8   Relational interdependence and triadic co-evolution   141

9   Constructing networks   152

10 The multi-process analysis   166

    Concluding remarks. Beyond psychotherapy   181
    Index   186

Series Editors Foreword

Charlotte Burck and Gwyn Daniel

We are so pleased to be able to introduce this book, *Psychotherapeutic Competencies. Techniques, Relationships, and Epistemology in Systemic Practice,* which we think is a rich treasure trove of resources for trainers, trainees, supervisors, and experienced therapists alike.

Laura Fruggeri, Francesca Balestra, and Elena Venturelli, a team of experienced clinician researchers, focus in a profound way on the complexities of interactional processes in therapy, filling theoretical gaps in our systemic knowledges. Their innovative drawing of distinctions of the different therapeutic competencies – technical competency, relational competency, epistemological competency, and expertise in multi-process analysis presents a new, refreshingly rigorous, and illuminating systemic framework for the field. The book is deeply informed by the authors' extensive clinical and training experiences and underpinned by process research studies. The authors unpack the complexities of the intrapersonal, interpersonal, social, cultural, and institutional processes of psychotherapy with a clarity that will enable trainee therapists, their trainers, and experienced therapists to easily apply these to their own clinical practice.

Commencing with a thought-provoking review of the common factors in psychotherapy, the authors go on to expand these generic features and elaborate the specific aspects of the practice of systemic psychotherapy.

The authors achieve elegantly, and as if effortlessly, a rare combination of research findings, observational analysis of interactional patterns, and creative reflective practice. By illustrating what is required of therapists at each of the technical, relational, and epistemological levels and in moving between levels, the authors invite therapists to critically reflect on their own thinking and their therapeutic assumptions.

One of the delights of this book is that it continually reminds us of the extraordinary contribution of the Milan group of therapists, of which Laura Fruggeri and her co-authors are such distinguished successors. The work of Gregory Bateson is central, as it was with the original Milan group, although here the authors frame his contribution as being social constructionist – concerned with social actors negotiating social realities – and profoundly relevant to contemporary therapists for whom social and cultural contexts are crucial. In discussing epistemological competencies, the authors provide wonderful descriptions of therapists and families negotiating together from the positions of their varying "local epistemologies" as they navigate through social worlds that constantly require of us a rethinking of assumptions.

One of the treasures of this book is the way that the theoretical descriptions are brilliantly interwoven with clinical material; just as one thinks "I'd like an example here", one is invariably provided. This interlinking of theoretical concepts and clinical examples is the hallmark of a book that will be invaluable for therapists and trainers of therapists alike.

We have no doubt that the book will fulfil its intention as a superb resource for training courses and will also open up the riches of systemic thinking and practice to those unfamiliar and less conversant with the field. We can also guarantee, as we ourselves experienced, that it has a huge amount to teach all of us as systemic psychotherapists and practitioners.

We are delighted to have this valuable book in our series.

Foreword

Imelda McCarthy

A renewed emphasis on therapeutic competencies in systemic practice

This book by Laura Fruggeri, Francesca Balestra and Elena Venturelli is a response to a growing call for a resurgence in systemic literature and trainings that emphasise therapeutic skill sets and competencies. At the outset of the systemic family therapy field, there was a huge focus on "how to" practice. With time and the advent of a more theoretically inclined social constructionism, an emphasis on skill sets declined in favour of a more dialogically focused quality of therapeutic interactions. I am so pleased to be able to hail this work as a bringing together of both skill sets *and* the importance of relational intelligence within therapy practices. Both are necessary and urgently called for in this time of neoliberal cutbacks and questionable evidence-based tick boxes.

I have long admired the work of Laura Fruggeri and her colleagues at the Centro Bolognese di Terapia della Famiglia. They have the gift of seamlessly bringing together the above concerns in the field of systemic practice. Throughout the book, clear and simple case examples are offered to introduce initiates to the thinking and practice of systemic practice and as a refresher for those with long years of experience. The case examples, of course, also act as a lead in to thinking about the issues being elaborated in each of the chapters.

Complexity, rigour, and imagination

Reading the list of contents, I was excited at the prospect of so much practice wisdom alongside what I imagined would also be a strong research, theoretical, and philosophical orientation. The central siting of the therapeutic relationship, the contexts of both clients and therapists together with the "person" of the therapist as experienced by clients are headlined as necessary indicators of good therapy. Thus, concentrating on research of what works in co-creating positive results in therapeutic practice is highlighted as a necessity in the toolkits of therapists. This takes a multi-dimensional approach to therapeutic relationships/ alliances, methods, and a therapist's way of being in the relationship. It is not an anything-goes approach but one which values good training and skill but not at the expense of the quality of therapist–client/family relationship and a very human way of being in the process. Now this is what marks this book out from many others. It has all the components brought together into a coherent whole. In the 1990s, there was a movement in family therapy away from a "methods and techniques" orientation in practice. Dialogue and reflexivity came to stand for method and technique, except in this writer's experience, most new therapists did not really know what that meant or how to work with it in sessions with complex client requests. In a way the new approaches seemed to both highlight complexity but at the expense of a rigorous practice approach. A systemic approach always incorporates complexity and many of the early pioneering work, including the work of Laura Fruggeri and her colleagues, showed students and workshop attendees HOW TO hold complexity together with tried and tested systemic conversations, dialogical and communicational skills. These skills not only showed through the conversations of therapy but also in the ways of thinking about individuals and their families in the context of their relationships AND in the context of the larger socio-political policies and practices in their environments.

This makes psychotherapy a complex mix of levels that include the intrapersonal, the interpersonal, the social, the cultural, and the institutional fields. Therefore, our competencies need to be honed to each of these levels, often simultaneously, within conversations with clients. Hence, the skill and practice of self-reflexivity is a crucial centre piece within these therapeutic competencies. How am I formed and "de-formed" within the contexts I am part of and interacting with? Systemic therapy has always been about seeing the presented problem as both relationally AND contextually situated. While this might make sense, the authors point out that these competencies in self-reflexivity are not natural. They need to be learned and practiced with both imagination and rigour. I would echo strongly this assertation.

Second-order reflexivities

The invitation of this work is to constantly think about how one is able to be a participant/observer, both WITHIN the therapeutic relationship and its context in a disposition of curiosity. Here Systemic practices (contextually reflexive observations, actions, and interactions) are allied with Social Constructionism (the co-construction of change) and Dialogical approaches (stressing collaboration and negotiation). As such, the concepts of "hypothesizing" and "questioning" are re-dressed as intersubjective processes between clients and therapists with due attention to issues of reflective power, inequality, and colonization in the therapeutic encounter. Questions are not just a one-way street within a top-down inquiry but are also exploratory, interventive, and transforming for both clients and therapists as they observe, articulate, and respond.

The therapeutic alliance is seen on two levels, the quality of the relationship between therapists and clients and the co-construction of meaning within the relationship. To this I would humbly suggest that this book also elaborates a third element of the alliance, and that is the synergistic nature of the behavioural interactions in sessions. So, while co-constructing a safe environment for individuals, couples, and families, a central part of synergetic intention is that "there will be no consequences for what they (clients) say during therapeutic encounters". I wonder how many of us take this as seriously as we ought to when we as therapists engage in sessions.

The book also explores the use of the SOFTA model (the System for Observing Family Therapy Alliances) as a tool for a constant self-reflexive monitoring, observation, and reporting of what is going on in therapist–client relationships and sessions. It is transtheoretical, multidimensional, and interpersonal in its construction. As such, this tool offers us an important, if not a crucial, resource on our own self-reflexive journeys with clients in context. This is especially so in the context of the importance of the client's perception of the therapeutic alliance. As with other competencies in this book, both the positives and limitations are also highlighted.

As the book progresses through relational competencies, which include acknowledgement of unintended consequences, seeing topics of conversation as contexts for relational competence, the authors stress that they see method and technique as being secondary to relational competence. The highlighting of the relational context as a guiding principle for therapists is important on the therapeutic path. However, this does not occlude that this, too, is also embedded in complex and interpenetrating socio-economic-political and cultural contexts. What I liked very much was the pointing towards possibilities of being seduced by the experience of therapy as a secure and safe space. While the systemic therapeutic relationship and space needs to build in safety in my experience given its complex nature, it also needs to maintain a healthy non-attachment to complete safety. This dilemma is nicely illustrated by the client who had to maintain a problematic profile in order for the therapy to continue. Therapy had become too much of a secure base and less of a diving platform that he could launch himself into a more preferred life.

Double vision

As the work progresses, the authors continually show how maintaining a double vision can manifest through technical and relational competencies in therapeutic practice. This double vision also relates to the process of what Bateson might refer to as abduction. This is when we see a similar pattern or parallel process emerging in two contexts, such as a couple pattern and a therapeutic pattern. The sections relating to this double vision and description towards the end of Chapter 4 are a must-read for any systemic therapist. They also function as a great lead into Chapters 5 and 6 on reflexivity, intersectionalities, personal epistemologies, and power.

In my own experience, this is the centre of what makes us systemic practitioners – an openness to our own (potential) biases, a willingness to explore different ways of seeing the world before us, and an ability to change our actions and interactions when called for. In other words, to practice complex thinking epistemologically, ontologically, and relationally.

One of practices that I value highly in systemic work is what the authors refer to as "divergent thinking". All therapy is offering "out-of-the-box" thinking in the service of clients (and indeed therapists), breaking free of habitual thinking, or what I call default modes (redundancies). Our loyalty to our own default modes can keep us very stuck as therapists and also only serve to maintain the problem that we are all trying to solve together. Curiosity, of course, is a superb antidote to being stuck in one's own premises or a hardened theoretical viewpoint, which can in turn lead to the abuse and colonization of a client's life and narrative [McCarthy 1990, 1991, 1994, 1995]. Being curious has the advantage that we can step away from our own or others' fixed ideas. In this stepping away from habitual or rigid theoretical modes of thinking, we become "decentred" in the authors' words. In this decentred mode, we are more fluidly placed to follow the stream of our client's thinking and rationale. Double description and multiple descriptions replace singular and linear prescriptions and proscriptions of a client's or family's life.

Co-evolution and co-creativity

Throughout the later sections of the book, we are reminded again and again of the importance of relational contexts in the life of our clients AND in our co-creative work with them. Without this we are shown through the case examples of how unless we can co-evolve together then we risk the identified client not being able to reach their goal and transform their lives in the way that they want. However, we are also invited to see beyond the immediate relational network to the broader support systems with whom the client and family interact. Circularity, inter-dependence and co-evolution are not just seen as intra-familial processes but also ones that encompass the client, family, therapist, and wider professional systems and networks of care. Time and time again we see the dangers of the lack of collaboration and co-ordination of a network of care in leading to a replication or mirroring of the patterns in the family. When this happens, we can see that fragmentation occurs with the risk of escalating symptomatology. Co-ordinated networks, on the other hand, recognize the complexity of the family/care systems and promote greater possibilities for the co-creation of coherent and shared treatment plans. A both/and circular frame replaces a dualistic linear frame for diagnoses, hypotheses, and conversational processes at all levels of the systems that we are both acting into and out of. The authors do not shy away from very difficult clinical scenarios, which included working with clients who are refugees and torture survivors and addressing the political and social contexts of resultant traumas, social prejudices, and changing population demographics. Hence, trauma is not individualized, pathologized, and decontextualized. These are not insignificant issues for all clinicians, especially in the light of the current pre-occupation with individualized accounts of trauma on social media and professional literature. Political, economic, social, and relational violence are matters of human rights and not just individualized psychological expressions.

As we read through the book the thread of the multi-connected contextualized "self" is stressed over and over again with illustrations from theory and practice. This applies to the "self" of clients and also therapists. The latter are invited into a rigorous application and demonstration of epistemology, theory, and practice. As systemic therapists there is a great stress on multi-dimensional competencies for basic self-reflection through self reflexivities in ongoing interactions at all levels – individual, relational, and social. The basic orientation is one of collaborative intent, where curiosity, openness, and flexibility are hallmarks of a respectful and non-instructive position (except when invited by clients to be otherwise in specific situations). This of course means a constant inner and outer awareness in dialogue with each other all the time. Curiosity, respect, and openness mean that we are also ready to change direction and hypotheses in service of clients. In other words, while there is a call to rigour there is also a call towards imagination and co-creativity.

One of the highlights of this book for me is that it presents the material in a way that is not only useful to clinicians at all levels but also that it can be used as training material for thinking, reflecting, and practicing systemic therapies. We are constantly re-minded about the importance of relational competencies, ethical practices, and awareness of one's own premises in order to have a clearer view of and way of potentiating, what the authors call, a multi-processual and co-evolutionary approach. Given the multi-cultural nature of the societies that most of us live in these days, such ongoing attention and diligence to our practice is of the highest ethical concern. This is no less true for all of those who live on the margins of our societies. For too long, our European and Anglo/American standards of so-called "normal" living have held sway in the face of very different cultural traditions of many of the clients and families we see. This book calls for a constant deconstruction of such potential colonial practices. This facilitates learning and illumination from the margins [McCarthy and Byrne 2019] to light our paths. Allowing clients and families to guide us into their particular life and relational spaces is both a privilege and an ethical imperative. I love the Batesonian thread running through this great text in the guises of abduction, non-instructive interaction, second-order reflexivities, circularity, and co-evolution. As such, the genius of Gianfranco Cecchin and Luigi Boscolo break through constantly as a reminder of the origins of the inspiration Italian systemic authors of this book.

References

McCarthy, I.C. [1990], *Paradigms lost: re-membering her-stories and other invalid subjects*, Journal of Contemporary Family Therapy, 12, pp. 427–437.

McCarthy, I.C. [1991], *Colonial sentences and just subversions: the potential for love and abuse in therapeutic encounters*, Feedback, 3, pp. 3–7.

McCarthy, I.C. [1994], *Abusing norms: welfare families and a fifth province stance*, in, I.C. McCarthy (ed.), *Poverty and social exclusion a special issue of human systems*, 5, ¾, pp. 229–239 (chosen as one of the influential papers over 10 years of Human Systems)

McCarthy, I.C. [1995], *Serving those in poverty: a benevolent colonisation?*, in, J. van Lawick and M. Sanders (eds.), *Gender and beyond*, Amsterdam, LS Books.

McCarthy, I. and Byrne, N. [2019], *A fifth province approach to intracultural issues in an irish context: marginal illuminations*, in, M. McGoldrick and K. Hardy (eds.), *Revisioning family therapy*, 3rd Edition, New York, Guilford Press.

Preface

The idea of writing this book came about during the peer supervisory sessions we have carried out over the last few years, both among ourselves and with other colleagues. The various occasions in which we have been able to reflect on the reasons for a therapeutic impasse have gradually stimulated in us the desire to be able to systematize what emerged, reconnecting it to the different areas of psychotherapeutic competency that were highlighted from time to time. Areas that only partly had to do with the technical dimension of therapy, i.e., with the tools of the therapeutic model, but which instead concerned the ethical, aesthetic, and reflexive dimensions of therapy. In other words, the values involved in the encounter between therapist and clients, the relational and interactive forms that the encounter generates, and the need for the therapists to be aware of their own position in the process.

Psychotherapy is a profession that undoubtedly implies knowledge of theories, procedures, and methodologies; it implies a technical competency that is situated in a specific model, in a conceptual framework that defines the clinician's universe of investigation, the conception of distress, the methods used to collect information, and the methods of intervention. However, the relationship between therapist and client, and the context in which this relationship takes shape, are not simply the background of the psychotherapeutic intervention, but the very plot through which it develops.

The concept of psychotherapy at the basis of this book is that of a meeting between people, which develops in a dialogical form in a socio–cultural–institutional context, with the aim of helping those who request it to overcome the conditions that produce psychological discomfort. This is a complex process involving different levels (individual, interpersonal, social) and requiring different skills. First, the ability to build and analyze the relationship and the interactive process of production of meanings that the therapist and clients contribute to build. But also, the therapists' ability to decentre and analyze situations from different points of view, recognizing the client's subjectivity and taking responsibility for their own premises. These are skills that help therapists to regain a generative position when technical competency no longer effectively supports their work. Moreover, the contextual aspect of psychotherapies is an element that is fundamental in the outcome of the intervention itself, which in fact takes on meanings also in relation to the interpersonal, cultural, and social life contexts of clients and to the institutional network within which therapy is conducted.

The chapters of this book are therefore dedicated to the conceptual tools that nourish and develop these competencies, which we define as second level since they concern the construction and monitoring of the therapeutic process.

This volume is intended as a sourcebook for colleagues in training, to help them orient themselves in the complexity that the encounter with the Other involves and invite them to develop the competencies here described, but also for colleagues already working in the profession, who want to reflect on their own professional development.

Laura Fruggeri
Francesca Balestra
Elena Venturelli

Acknowledgements

The writing of this book would not have been possible without encounters with the people who relied on us, allowing us to enter their life stories and grow with them. Our first thanks, therefore, go to all the clients we have met, directly or indirectly. The richness of the stories reported in the text is also the result of the exchange with our colleagues Anna Castellucci, Andrea Davolo, and Monica Sparamonti, to whom we express our gratitude for having shared with us their reflection on some cases. We thank Federico Ferrari and Jimmy Ciliberto for agreeing to write the text for some boxes. We are grateful to Marina Everri for helping with the translation of some chapters. We are also grateful to Gail Simon for the encouraging interest shown in our work and for permission to use some material published by Everything is Connected Press. Thanks are due to Maurizio Marzari and all the colleagues at the Centro Bolognese di Terapia della Famiglia, with whom we have been sharing experiences, ideas, and reflections, as well as our training history, for years.

This book is more than a translation of the original Italian book. Thanks to the precious editing and advice of Gwyn Daniel and Charlotte Burk, we have had the possibility to frame the book further in terms of an international multicultural professional context. Finally, our gratitude goes to Imelda McCarthy for supporting the project of translating the book in English since the beginning and for doing us the honor of writing the foreword.

Laura Fruggeri
Francesca Balestra
Elena Venturelli

Introduction: specific and common factors of psychotherapy

Psychotherapy as a social construction

Psychotherapy can be considered a cooperative enterprise deriving from the negotiation and creation of stories shared between therapists and clients within a specific context and time.

The dance metaphor has been used to describe interpersonal processes, and as such, it is appropriate to describe psychotherapeutic processes, since they entail the coordination of actions autonomously generated, while being connected in a way that shapes visible interactive forms. In this sense, the minimal unit of meaning and analysis is not a single action; rather, it is a sequence of actions. As Norén and Linell [2007] point out, the meaning of an action can be better understood from the observation of the response made to that action. The usefulness of a therapeutic intervention cannot be deduced from the therapists' evaluation of their intervention; it can rather be inferred from the client's response. As reported by Schegloff [2007], actions performed during an interactive process can be *context-shaped,* namely constructed as a response to precedent actions, and *context-renewing,* since every action creates the context for subsequent actions. In this sense, elaborating further on the dance metaphor, therapists should know the basic moves, but they should also be able to improvize since what the therapists plan to say changes in the very moment they say it [Escott 2011]. In other words, the therapists need to modulate and adjust their thoughts and language according to the feedback received by their clients.

Social constructionism has emphasized the process dimension of psychotherapy: psychotherapist and client are both actors acting according to their premises and to their different roles on the stage of the therapeutic encounter, with the aim to create a system in which the coordination between old and new information generates a new narrative [McNamee and Gergen 1992; Penn and Frankfurt 1994; Fruggeri 2012].

System and *context* are the other key words of our approach to therapy. These two notions refer to the awareness of the multiple levels implied in the process of psychotherapy. They invite reflection on how the dance between therapists and clients occurs within wider socio-cultural-political-institutional contexts, which affect individual responses as well as intimate relations;

DOI: 10.4324/9781003278092-1

moreover, they invite exploration on "how change in one part of the system has transformational influence in unexpected ways and places immediately and/or elsewhere" [McCarthy and Simon 2016, p. XIII].

The complexity of the multiple aspects that are implied in a therapeutic process, is empirically documented by the research on factors affecting the positive outcome of therapies.

Research on specific and common factors of psychotherapy

The international community of clinicians and researchers agrees on the fact that psychotherapy works. The positive impact of psychotherapy can be found in a variety of situations and contexts: psychological treatments are effective for children, adults, and elderly people; for individuals, families, and couples; in private practices or in public centres; in emergency and compulsory treatments – and in many other situations. The question as to whether psychotherapy works has now found convergent and convincing positive answers from the literature. But other questions, concerning "how" and "why" psychotherapy works, are nowadays animating the debate among professionals of different orientations. On these questions, researchers have long been divided.

Some scholars have focused their investigation on techniques and tools provided by the various therapeutic models, that is, on those factors defined as "specific" because they characterize a given theoretical-methodological approach. Research on specific factors assumes that techniques play a central role in the success of therapy. This type of investigation is aimed at demonstrating the validity of a particular therapeutic model, and at detecting clinical situations in which one model proves to be valid or more valid than others. The investigation has sometimes comparative purposes, i.e., it questions which model or models are most effective in general or in treating specific psychopathological situations.

Other researchers have instead paid attention to the link between the positive psychotherapeutic outcome and a series of factors detectable in all therapeutic contexts regardless of the adopted model; namely, the quality of the relationship between the clinician and client, the characteristics of the client, the context, and the therapist. These elements are unrelated to the adopted theoretical and methodological model, and as such are defined as "non-specific or common factors". In this case, the researchers shift the focus away from the efficacy of the techniques and question instead "whether" and "to what extent" factors that can transversely be found in all therapeutic processes affect the positive outcome of psychotherapy.

Over the years, the two different approaches have given rise to interesting results and reflections.

Research on the role of specific factors in psychotherapeutic outcomes

In the early 1990s, researchers who addressed the empirical validation of psychotherapies focused on techniques. The complex studies conducted with the aim of empirically proving the efficacy of psychotherapeutic treatments achieved results that were particularly relevant to psychotherapy, as they clearly established its efficacy and demonstrated that it can be the treatment of choice for specific disorders [Chambless and Hollon 1998; Chambless and Ollendick 2001; American Psychological Association 2006]. Through rigorous experimental procedures, the empirically supported treatments movement has emphasised the importance of testing psychotherapies with the twofold aim of 1) providing data to support the therapeutic validity of the various models and their techniques[1]; and 2) operationalizing and standardizing the different models. These studies built upon research data to draw the boundaries that operationally define what a given therapeutic model consists of, to develop protocols that can provide clinicians with a guide to effectively respond to clients' needs. In other words, the focus on the specific technical factors of the various therapeutic models has prompted the clinical and scientific community to operationally define the therapeutic models, indicating their healing properties and identifying guidelines (manuals) that allow clinicians to be as rigorous as possible in applying a model whose validity has been scientifically proven. In this light, operationalization and standardization of treatments are at the basis of a virtuous circle leading to the achievement of a positive therapeutic outcome, as they allow for training therapists in rigorous use of the techniques, maximizing the possibility for controlling the consistency with the model. However, this very concept of clinical effectiveness based on the standardization of variables has led to a series of objections.

Testing the empirical validity of a treatment entails a series of methodological premises that are functional to the success of a clinical trial, but cannot be considered "neutral", since the structure of the research design conveys specific assumptions concerning psychological processes, clients, and the therapeutic process itself [Westen, Novotny and Thompson-Brenner 2004]. The main critique to this line of research is epistemological and concerns the reductionism of the very notion of psychotherapy underlying the investigation: a conception of psychotherapy as a mechanically and a-contextually applied technique [Roy-Chowdhury 2003]. This critique is grounded on methodology that is based on the randomization of patients' allocation and on the standardization of the considered variables. Indeed, outcome research involves the standardization of variables such as age, severity of symptoms, level of clients' functioning, degree of therapists' experience and competence, length of therapy, and adherence to the model. Also, it is necessary to establish an agreement on what will be considered an outcome, on what will be considered a change, and on what instruments will measure it [Davey *et al.* 2012]. Most importantly, research on model validity implies controlling the independent variable, namely the psychotherapy itself, to test the cause–effect relation between therapeutic intervention and outcome. This requires the operationalization and standardization of treatment, and manuals meet this need. However, the manualization of therapeutic interventions brings us back to the initial criticism concerning the reduction of psychotherapy to a mechanical and a-contextual application of techniques. But critiques go beyond the epistemological level. Research has shown that the variables affecting the positive outcome of a therapy are far from being homogeneous. Indeed, research data from both naturalistic studies and meta-analyses emphasize that the most effective treatments vary in duration from 1 to 2 years, and that clients treated with brief therapies are more likely to seek additional treatment over the next 12 to 24 months [Seligman 1995]. Similarly, an inconsistency can be found with respect to the presenting problem, which is usually only one in this type of research, the one diagnosed at the beginning of the treatment, whereas clinical practice shows that comorbidity and inter-connections between different psychological problems are the rule [Oldham *et al.* 1995; Newman *et al.* 1998; Westen, Novotny and Thompson-Brenner 2004]. It is known to all therapists how a symptomatology addressed in the early stages of a psychotherapeutic treatment can subsequently allow other issues to emerge, which then become the primary focus of therapy over time. The focus on the symptom rather than on the therapeutic process carries another bias: psychological problems are separated from the characteristics of the person presenting them, thereby ignoring research data that underline how different personality characteristics can moderate both the psychological problem and the response to psychotherapy treatment.

The emphasis on the epistemological and functional limitation of an approach that puts specific technical factors of psychotherapy at the core of the process of change, is not aimed at disregarding its contribution. We prefer to acknowledge the complexity of the therapeutic process, and we would like to offer a reflection on the multiplicity of aspects that characterize effective psychotherapies. In doing so, we build upon research on psychotherapy outcomes that take into account the "non-specific" factors, which are "common" across all theoretical-technical models.

Investigation into the role of non-specific or common factors in psychotherapeutic outcomes

Psychotherapy is both an application of methodological and technical principles, and the development of a relationship between individuals. Starting from this consideration, several studies have shifted the attention to factors related to the psychotherapeutic situation, showing over the years how the outcome is only partially determined by the use of a specific technique or of a therapeutic approach in relation to a given symptomatology, and how relational and contextual factors seem to be involved in the success of a psychotherapy [Luborsky, Singer and Luborsky 1975; Frank 1976; Lambert 1992; Hubble, Duncan and Miller 1999; Wampold 2001; Sprenkle and Blow 2004]. A rigorous review of empirical research on psychotherapy outcomes conducted by Lambert [1992] found that elements linked to the client's history and context (i.e., extra-therapeutic factors) have the highest percentage of impact on therapeutic improvement (40%), followed by the quality of the relationship created between clients and therapists during the intervention (30%). The therapist's approach and the procedures associated with it have only a 15% influence on the outcome, as do the placebo factors and the client's positive expectation of the treatment, which also account for 15%. Research on the relationship between psychotherapy outcomes and non-specific factors overturns the perspective that identifies the driving force of change in the type of approach adopted. Indeed, the common factors model introduces the idea that any bona fide[2] treatment can be effective if it is able to convey a set of relational conditions considered necessary for change [Laska, Gurman and Wampold 2014]. They include: a positive emotional bond between client and therapist; a therapeutic context perceived as safe; an intervention that provides credible explanations and viable options to overcome specific difficulties; and involvement in the therapist's proposed intervention that allows the client to make adaptive changes in relation to the presented difficulties.

Within the study of non-specific factors, further investigation has been conducted on how clients' and therapists' characteristics may influence the therapeutic outcome. As to clients characteristics, research data have provided evidence of an aspect that all clinicians experience: the therapeutic relationship and the type of treatment that is provided must consider the peculiarities of each client and therefore adapt to them [Norcross and Wampold 2011]. Over the years, the client's characteristics have been considered mainly from the point of view of the presented problem, in search of the most effective match between the problem and the treatment. However, considering the client only in terms of clinical problem is an incomplete choice, which does not consider how other variables may distinguish one client from another and thus have an impact on the treatment. The goal of improving the effectiveness of therapeutic interventions by adapting them to the transdiagnostic characteristics of the clients led to interesting results. For instance, research indicates that clients' preferences that may influence the conclusion of a therapy both in terms of a drop-out and a positive outcome include: the attributes of the therapist (degree of experience and cultural background), the kind of treatment (behavioural or psychodynamic approach, counselling or psychotherapy), and the actions performed during the therapeutic process (a therapist who is more active or quieter, an individual or a group therapy) [Swift, Callahan and Vollmer 2011]. Clients who display high levels of oppositionality are more likely to respond to non-directive treatments [Beutler *et al.* 2011]. Tailoring the therapeutic stance to the clients' state of awareness of their problem increases the chances of successfully completing therapy. Namely, a Socratic therapeutic stance that fosters insight is more likely to be helpful when clients have little awareness of their problems or are still trying to define the outlines of their difficulties, whereas a counselling or coaching stance would be more effective in a more action-oriented phase [Prochaska and Norcross 2001]. In summary, these data demonstrate that a positive outcome is achievable insofar as the therapeutic encounter succeeds in activating the client's self-healing potential; this kind of assessment can only be made through an observation and analysis of the therapeutic relationship that has been established or is about to be established, and of the context that this relationship creates with a specific client.

Therapist characteristics are also considered as non-specific factors independent of the technical model. Such a consideration refers to the evidence that some clinicians achieve better results than other colleagues while offering the same type of treatment from a technical viewpoint. According to the studies that have been conducted on this topic, the most effective therapists are able to create a good alliance with a greater variety of clients; they have good interpersonal skills; they are flexible, open, respectful, trustworthy, and interested in the client; they provide explanations for the problem that are acceptable to the client, i.e., in line with the client's premises, values, and culture; they are not "culturally arrogant", i.e., they do not impose their beliefs on the clients, they remain attentive to what the clients bring; they are self-confident and self-reflective at the same time, i.e., capable of questioning their own work; they monitor their clients' change by discussing it with them; they are aware of their own internal processes and emotions and do not let them unwittingly interfere with the therapeutic process, but they are able to use them deliberately for clinical purposes; they exercise their therapeutic skills also in activities that take place outside the clinical setting [Ackerman and Hilsenroth 2003; Wampold and Carlson 2011; Wampold 2015; Norcross and Lambert 2018]. These aspects are very important as they define the set of skills that therapists should implement to be effective with their clients. Given that the impact of the therapist on the outcome of psychotherapy, the so-called "therapist effect", influences at least 5–8% of the outcome [Barkham *et al.* 2017], the above aspects should be placed at the heart of psychotherapists' training; nevertheless, they are often ignored by best practice guidelines, and not explicitly included in training courses.

Yet, over the years the common factor model and its clinical implications were not devoid of criticism. The main concern refers to the risk of weakening, or even worse discrediting, the different treatment models. Research evidence demonstrating that the same clinical problem can be addressed with equally positive outcomes by adopting different therapeutic approaches [Imber *et al.* 1990; Stiles *et al.* 2008; American Psychological Association 2013] has led the most radical proponents of the common factors approach to endorse the paradox of equivalence – known as "the Dodo's verdict"[3] [Rosenzweig 1936] – according to which all psychotherapies are equally effective. If literally taken, this stance is dangerous because it could convey the message that it does not matter what one does in therapy, or that highly validated therapies can be equated with less structured treatments such as counselling or relaxation techniques. Due to highlighting these pitfalls, a more moderate approach has emerged in the scientific community – one that does not deny the importance of specific clinical models, but rather emphasizes how other aspects, including those related to common factors, contribute to the therapeutic process by enhancing the techniques [Laska, Gurman and Wampold 2014]. Such considerations support a recalibration of the impact that the therapeutic relationship may have on the therapeutic outcome. While in the past some have argued that the therapeutic relationship would be sufficient to produce change [Patterson 1984], today even those who emphasize the importance of common factors are aware that although the quality of the therapeutic relationship is an element that has a profound effect on the success of therapy, there are many other elements that contribute to the achievement of this result. It should be noted that stressing the importance of common factors in relation to the therapeutic outcome does not lead to the assumption that therapists can do "whatever they want" from a technical point of view; it rather leads to reflection on how to improve the therapist's competence so that it is not reduced to a simplistic application of techniques, procedures, and protocols. A further point of criticism raised against the common factors approach concerns its alleged non-scientific nature, imputed to the difficulty of operationalizing and standardizing the variables involved. In response to this criticism, the American Psychological Association's Society for the Advancement of Psychotherapy (Division 29, created in 1999) focused on the empirical investigation of the therapeutic relationship dimensions. The collected research data document how therapeutic alliance, empathy, shared purpose, collaboration, and emotional connection between client and therapist are all elements that actively contribute to the achievement of a positive outcome [Norcross 2001; Norcross and Lambert 2018]. As we will discuss in more detail in Chapter 3, knowledge about the therapeutic alliance is the proof that even common factors can be manualized and taught [Escudero 2012].

For a long time, the term "evidence-based practice" has been used as a synonym for "empirically supported treatments", implicitly conveying the idea that only practices that have been subjected to randomized controlled clinical trials can be considered scientifically valid and thus appropriately and rigorously usable. However, the studies on the therapeutic relationship and on common factors, which have documented in a richer and more systematic way the weight of these factors on the therapeutic outcome, have increasingly contributed to expanding the meaning of evidence-based practice. It includes all research data that enable clinicians to achieve the best possible therapeutic outcome, that is, everything in a therapeutic system that leads to a positive outcome [Sprenkle and Blow 2004]. Within an evidence-based clinical practice, the focus on non-specific factors of therapy allows the implementation of process research methodologies, thus focusing on what happens during the therapeutic encounter. Therefore, the analysis is both on the "effective technique", and on what results in a positive effect for that client, involved in a relationship with that therapist, within a given context. In an equally rigorous way, by adopting this lens therapists can also begin to ask themselves about the context they are contributing to create as they apply model-specific techniques (see Chapter 4).

Towards complex models

Research on specific and non-specific factors has contributed to the identification of different components that come into play in the therapeutic process as well as documenting their impact on the successful outcome of the treatment.

However, it is important to note that techniques, relational factors, and participants' characteristics, when considered independently, do not have much impact on client improvement [Castonguay and Beutler 2006]. The debate on which elements of psychotherapy are relevant for a positive outcome can no longer focus on the dominance of one factor at the expense of others, but it must be oriented towards providing maps through which the complex relationship between specific and non-specific variables can be described.

An interesting attempt to integrate these different components has been proposed by Fife and colleagues [2014] with a meta-model called "Therapeutic Pyramid" (see Figure 0.1), which considers the interconnection of 3 factors: technique, therapeutic alliance, and the therapist's way of being. The technical dimension refers to the knowledge and use of specific therapeutic approaches and related methodologies. Although necessary, technical proficiency is not sufficient for therapeutic success: clinical models are implemented through the relationship between client and therapist. In Fife and colleagues' model, the relational dimension is proposed in terms of therapeutic alliance, defined as the quality and strength of the collaborative relationship between the client and therapist that is established regardless of the therapy model used [Horvath 2001].

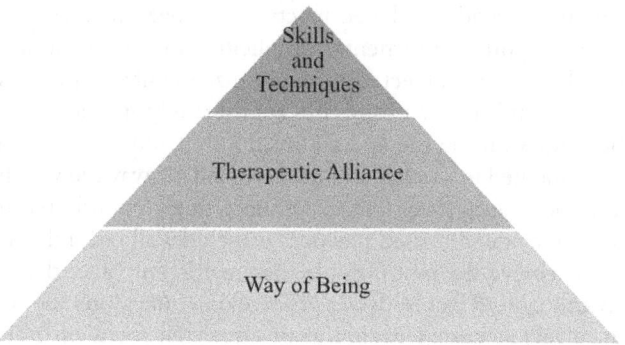

Figure 0.1 The therapeutic pyramid [Fife *et al.* 2014].

The hierarchical structure of the model suggests that the technique placed at the top of the pyramid is effective when it is grounded in a good alliance between the client and therapist, which in turn depends on how the therapists position themself towards their clients. The therapist's way of being, placed at the base of the pyramid, refers to the attitude that therapists have towards clients in the here and now of therapy. Through attitude, tone of voice, and word choice, therapists can make clients feel like unique human beings who deserve to be listened to and not judged, or, conversely, objectify them by making them feel like "clinical cases" to be placed in the right diagnostic category, limiting the recognition of their uniqueness. The way of being, as intended in this model, leads to a reflection on the therapists' ability to "see" the other, that is, to work on their own self, to be able to decentre and grasp the reality that clients bring. By describing the therapeutic process in this way, we can see that the lower levels of the pyramid support and influence the higher levels: therapists who value the client's uniqueness by decentring themself to understand the client's point of view will make the construction of a positive alliance more likely, creating a relational context within which they practice the technical expertise with greater success by choosing the most suitable methodologies for that specific situation. On the contrary, a good technical and theoretical proficiency, that is to say the ability to master the tools of the clinical approach, does not necessarily result in establishing a positive relationship with the client or in adopting a position of acceptance of the client's experiences. The outcomes of the research described here underline the importance for clinicians to reflect on the complexity of therapeutic skills they keep in their "toolbox".

Psychotherapeutic competency as a multi-faceted construct

Psychotherapy, as it emerges from the research on its effectiveness, implies different levels of intrapersonal, interpersonal, social, cultural, and institutional processes so that a therapist devoted to this complex professional practice needs to learn and practice different skills concerning different aspects of "doing therapy". In this sense, therapeutic competency can be represented by a prismatic image whose different and interconnected faces are: the ability to use one's skills to create a generative conversational space (technical competency); the ability to build a good alliance with clients and to participate in the creation of transformative relational contexts (relational competency); the ability to know how to change point of view, decentring in order to grasp the client's point of view and practicing self-reflexivity to become aware of one's own premises (epistemological competency); and the ability to grasp how people's life contexts affect their system of meanings, their actions, and the development of therapies (context sensitivity or acknowledgment of the context).

Technical competency as a dialogical construction of a shared symbolic space. Within the systemic model, the idea of the context as a matrix of meanings applied to the analysis of psycho-pathological phenomena and to the psychotherapeutic setting has introduced a revolution in the way of considering clinical categories such as symptoms, diagnosis, and treatment, redefining them in relational terms. The symptom is not treated as an expression of individual dysfunctions, but it is instead assumed as information concerning the entire network of relationships in which the person is inserted; the diagnosis is not the attribution of pathological categories to a single individual, but it refers to the functioning of a group; the therapeutic intervention is not based on the analysis of intrapsychic processes, but on the observation of the interactive dynamics and patterns of the whole family group and aims at modifying the context within which the discomfort has emerged and is maintained. The framework within which the therapists get to "know" the client's situation is the dialogue they have with the client since the first meeting. From a socio-constructivist point of view, in fact, the investigation that the therapist carries out can be seen both as a collection of information and as an offer of information; through the questions, the therapist participates in the process of co-construction of an intersubjective reality that can be of the same type or different from the one that the clients and their significant system have built in their history/experience. In this sense, the psychotherapist's dialogical competency refers to the ability to conduct a collaborative conversation, co-generative of transformative processes. Being in a transformative dialogue with people requires presence and attention to the moment one is living, but if on the one hand each dialogue is unique, on the other hand, as we will describe in the chapters of the first part, there are specific elements, questions, and interventions that can generate and promote the flow of dialogue and in turn help to mobilize the resources of the persons and their network.

Relational competency: promoting and analysing intersubjectivity. The common factors approach identifies the therapeutic relationship as one of the elements that most affects the success of treatment. In the literature, the therapeutic relationship is often considered in terms of therapeutic alliance, that is, the quality and strength of the collaborative relationship between client and therapist, and the ability to negotiate treatment goals and tasks [Bordin 1979]. A positive therapist–client alliance is essential to achieve good results: clients' behaviours, in terms of listening, resistance to change, and even the interruption or not of the therapy will depend on the clients' perception of how much the therapist cares for them [Friedlander, Escudero and Heatherington 2006]. In this sense, the therapist must be able to both analyze the alliance and build it [Escudero and Friedlander 2017], also relying on the meta-analyses that identify which therapist actions promote the creation of a good relationship for the purpose of positive therapy outcome [Norcross and Lambert 2018]. However, the relational competency of the therapist is not limited to building and maintaining a positive relationship with the client, it also involves considering the ways in which therapists and clients participate in the construction of meanings during their encounter. Relational competency is thus expressed through the ability to analyze and understand the process of co-construction through which clients and therapists generate identities, relationships, and social worlds [Roy-Chowdhury 2006; Fruggeri 2012], that is, to capture the cooperative dance of therapists and clients in order to recognize, create, and maintain transformative relational contexts. Joint processes of construction are therefore not about how people participate in interaction, but rather what they do together [Shotter 1993]. In this sense, relational competency allows a constant understanding of the interactive process that develops with clients, and therefore puts the therapists in a position to monitor the therapeutic process as it unfolds, and to "adjust" their actions so as to contribute to the construction of interactive situations in which clients can develop their skills and find answers to their needs. These two aspects of relational competency – that is, the ability to read the therapeutic process regarding both the construction of the therapeutic alliance, and the interactive process of construction of meanings – will be treated in the chapters of the second part.

Epistemological competency: the ability to change point of view. Psychotherapists base their technical competency on therapeutic models learned in structured training courses; these models constitute their formal and conscious knowledge. However, psychotherapists do not act only on the basis of formal knowledge. Like all social actors, they share an informal common sense knowledge that often unconsciously guides them in their choices as much as their formal knowledge. Therefore, a therapist needs to develop an epistemological competency, i.e., the ability to reflect on one's personal, socially and culturally shared premises, and how these tend to construct actions during the therapeutic process. Self-reflexivity is not simply the ability to reflect on what one knows or observes, but on how one knows and "how knowing is done" [Bateson and Bateson 1987, p. 19]. This kind of self-reflection allows psychotherapists to question both the effect of their own scientific techniques and theories, and their own prejudices and implicit beliefs that inevitably underlie their actions and that can stiffen the analysis of situations and the interventions. Self-reflexivity is the condition of being able to change point of view when the perspective assumed introduces rigidity into the system. But epistemological competency does not only concern the therapist's way of knowing. Cecchin [1987] invites therapists to develop an interest in the way clients make sense of their experiences and, therefore, to raise questions before reaching a conclusion, asking oneself, for example, from which point of view that particular behaviour can make sense. This is a decentring activity that puts the therapist in a position to connect with clients starting from "where they are" to help them move towards new perspectives. Self-reflexivity and decentring are the elements through which epistemological competency is practiced to protect psychotherapists from the iatrogenic effects deriving from the rigidity of their own model of reference [Cecchin, Lane and Ray 1992] and from a practice unconsciously oriented by prejudices, common sense, and naturalized beliefs sometimes stronger, just because they are unconscious, than professional knowledge [Bianciardi and Telfener 2014; Fruggeri 2015]. As we explain in the third part of the volume, self-reflexivity and decentring are not natural skills; they must be learned and practiced methodically.

Acknowledging the context: the social dimension of psychotherapy. Acknowledging the context concerns the therapist's awareness of operating in a broad environment that goes beyond the therapy room. An intervention cannot be considered therapeutic a priori, but only within the intertwining of meaning systems and interactions that characterizes the clients' relationships with their own system and those between them and the therapist [Rober 2017]. Acknowledging the context orients terapists to question the meaning that their intervention with clients takes on within the relationship between them and their significant others in their context of belonging; this allows the therapists to organize their intervention not simply on the basis of what they believe to be useful and developmental for the client, but on the basis of what they believe to be useful and developmental for the client as a component of a wider meaningful system. Following the developmental psychologist Bronfenbrenner [1979], we can indeed say that only what is evolutionary in the context of a person's meaningful relationships is also evolutionary for the person.

The concepts of "interdependence" and "co-evolution" also apply to those complex situations in which people are taken in charge by a network of services. To trigger evolutionary processes, it is necessary that the therapeutic system considers the interventions of the different agencies as closely interconnected. This implies for practitioners to consider themself as "part of" and therefore in relation with all the other components of the working group [Fruggeri *et al.* 1991; Asen, Dawson and McHugh 2001]. Developing this competency allows therapists to analyze the complexity within which people are embedded without running the risk of parcelling out and/or making their interventions useless. In Rober's words [2017, p. 37], the psychotherapist must pay attention to connecting "with the resources of the client and his/her social context; and give enough room to these resources in the therapeutic process. Respect these resources and seek ways to collaborate with them".

But acknowledging the context means also being aware of the intertwining between psychological distress and quality of social relationships, underlining how intrapersonal aspects are connected with inter-individual ones, and with socio-economic-cultural-institutional conditions, such as gender, power, poverty, and inequality, urging psychotherapists to make a critical reflection on how they, in carrying out their interventions, guided by models that ignore the differences created by social relations, may inadvertently and unconsciously contribute to reconstructing such differences. These themes will be addressed in the fourth part.

Notes

1 An example of this type of systemic orientation is the work by Stratton *et al.* [2010]. The European project coordinated by Stratton is based on previous research that found systemic family therapy to be the treatment of choice in cases of depression [Leff *et al.* 2000] and in cases of substance abuse [Joanning *et al.* 1992]. Systemic family therapy has also proved to be highly effective in recent investigations for the treatment of both adults and children [Carr 2018; 2019].

2 The term "bona fide treatment" refers to a treatment that is widely practiced in the clinical setting, with a recognized theoretical structure and empirical basis [Wampold 2001].

3 The term was coined referring to an episode from Lewis Carroll's *Alice in Wonderland*. Alice and other characters find themselves taking part in a race that has no fixed duration or route. When anyone stops and asks curiously who came first, the Dodo replies, "Everybody won, everybody has to get a prize".

References

Ackerman, S.J. and Hilsenroth, M.J. [2003], *A review of therapist characteristics and techniques positively impacting the therapeutic alliance*, in Clinical Psychology Review, 23, 1, pp. 1–33.

American Psychological Association [2006], *Evidence-based practice in psychology: APA presidential task force on evidence-based practice*, in American Psychologist, 61, 6, pp. 271–285

American Psychological Association [2013], *Recognition of psychotherapy effectiveness*, in Psychotherapy, 50, pp. 102–109.

Asen, E., Dawson, N. and McHugh, B. [2001], *Multiple family therapy: the Marlborough Model and its wider applications*, London, Karnac.

Barkham, M., Lutz, W., Lambert, M.J. and Saxon, D. [2017], *Therapist effects, effective therapists, and the law of variability*, in L. Castonguay and C. Hill (eds.), *How and why are some therapists better than others? Understanding therapist effects*, Washington DC, American Psychological Press, pp. 13–36.

Bateson, G. and Bateson, M.C. [1987], *Angels fear*, New York, Macmillan.

Beutler, L.E., Harwood, T.M., Michelson, A., Song, X. and Holman, J. [2011], *Resistance/reactance level*, in Journal of Clinical Psychology, 67, pp. 133–142.

Bianciardi, M. and Telfener, U. [2014], *Ricorsività in psicoterapia: riflessioni sulla pratica clinica*, Torino, Bollati Boringhieri.

Bronfenbrenner, U. [1979], *The ecology of human development*, Cambridge MA, Harvard University Press.

Bordin, E. [1979], *The generalizability of the psychoanalytic concept of the working alliance*, in Psychotherapy: Theory, Research and Practice, 16, pp. 252–260.

Carr, A. [2018], *Couple therapy, family therapy and systemic interventions for adult-focused problems: the current evidence base*, in Journal of Family Therapy, 40, 4, pp. 492–536.

Carr, A. [2019], *Family therapy and systemic interventions for child-focused problems: the current evidence base*, in Journal of Family Therapy, 41, 2, pp. 153–213.

Castonguay, L.G. and Beutler, L.E. [2006], *Principles of therapeutic change: a task force on participants, relationships, and techniques factors*, in Journal of Clinical Psychology, 62, 6, pp. 631–638.

Cecchin, G. [1987], *Hypothesizing, circularity, and neutrality revisited: an invitation to curiosity*, in Family Process, n. 26, 4, pp. 405–413.

Cecchin, G., Lane, G. and Ray, W.A. [1992], *Irreverence: a strategy for therapists' survival*, London, Karnac Books.

Chambless, D.L. and Hollon, S.D. [1998], *Defining empirically supported therapies*, in Journal of Consulting and Clinical Psychology, 66, 1, pp. 7–18.

Chambless, D.L. and Ollendick, T.H. [2001], *Empirically supported psychological interventions: controversies and evidence*, in Annual Review of Psychology, 52, 1, pp. 685–716.

Davey, M.P., Davey, A., Tubbs, C., Savla, J. and Anderson, S. [2012], *Second order change and evidence-based practice*, in Journal of Family Therapy, 34, 1, pp. 72–90.

Escudero, V. [2012], *Reconsidering the "heresy" of using treatment manuals*, in Journal of Family Therapy, 34, 1, pp. 106–113.

Escudero, V. and Friedlander, M.L. [2017], *Therapeutic alliances with families: empowering clients in challenging cases*, Berlin, Springer.

Escott, H. [2011], *Ciò che sarà detto e ciò che non si dice*, in Connessioni, 27, pp. 145–161.

Fife, S.T., Whiting, J.B., Bradford, K. and Davis, S. [2014], *The therapeutic pyramid: a common factors synthesis of techniques, alliance, and way of being*, in Journal of Marital and Family Therapy, 40, 1, pp. 20–33.

Frank, J.D. [1976], *Psychotherapy and the sense of mastery*, in R.L. Spitzer and D.F. Klein (eds.), *Evaluation of psychotherapies: behavior therapies, drug therapies, and their interactions*, Baltimore, Johns Hopkins University Press, pp. 47–56.

Friedlander, M.L., Escudero, V. and Heatherington, L. [2006], *Therapeutic alliances in couple and family therapy: an empirically informed guide to practice*, Washington DC, American Psychological Association.

Fruggeri, L. [2012], *Different levels of psychotherapeutic competence*, in Journal of Family Therapy, 34, pp. 91–105.

Fruggeri, L. [2015], *Il rischio iatrogeno in psicoterapia*, in Rivista Sperimentale di Freniatria, n. 3, pp. 105–116.

Fruggeri, L., Telfener, U., Castellucci, A., Marzari, M. and Matteini, M. [1991], *New systemic ideas from the Italian mental health movement*, London, Karnac Books.

Horvath, A.O. [2001], *The alliance*, in Psychotherapy, 38, 4, pp. 365–372.

Hubble, M.A., Duncan, B.L. and Miller, S. [1999], *The heart and soul of change*, Washington DC, American Psychological Association.

Imber, S.D., Pilkonis, P.A., Sotsky, S.M., Elkin, I., Watkins, J.T., Collins, J.F. and Glass, D.R. [1990], *Mode-specific effects among three treatments for depression*, in Journal of Consulting and Clinical Psychology, 58, 3, pp. 352–359.

Joanning, H., Quinn, W., Thomas, F. and Mullen, R. [1992], *Treating adolescent drug abuse: a comparison of family systems therapy, group therapy, and family drug education*, in Journal of Martial and Family Therapy, 18, 4, p. 345–356.

Lambert, M.J. [1992], *Psychotherapy outcome research: implications for integrative and eclectic therapists*, in J.C. Norcross and M.R. (eds.), *Handbook of psychotherapy integration*, Goldfried, New York, Basic Books, pp. 94–129.

Laska, K.M., Gurman, A.S. and Wampold, B.E. [2014], *Expanding the lens of evidence-based practice in psychotherapy: a common factors perspective*, in Psychotherapy, 51, 4, pp. 467–481.

Leff, J., Vearnals, S., Brewin, C.R., Wolff, G., Alexander, B., Asen E., Dayson, D., Jones, E., Chisholm, D. and Everitt, B. [2000], *The London Depression Intervention trial*, in British Journal of Psychiatry, 177, pp. 95–100.

Luborsky, L., Singer, B. and Luborsky, L. [1975], *Comparative studies of psychotherapy: is it true that "Everyone has won and all must have prizes?"*, in Archives of General Psychiatry, 32, pp. 995–1008.

Mc Carthy, I. and Simon, G. (eds.) [2016], *Systemic therapy as transformative practice*, Furnhill, UK, Everything is Connected Press.

Mc Namee, S. and Gergen, K. (eds.) [1992], *Therapy as social construction*, London, Sage.

Newman, D.L., Moffitt, T., Caspi, A. and Silva, P.A. [1998], *Comorbid mental disorders: implications for treatment and sample selection*, in Journal of Abnormal Psychology, 107, pp. 305–311.

Norén, K. and Linell, P. [2007], *Meaning potentials and the interaction between lexis and grammar. Some empirical substantiation*, in Pragmatics, 17, pp. 387–416.

Norcross, J.C. [2001], *Purposes, processes and products of the task force on empirically supported therapy relationships*, in Psychotherapy: Theory, Research, Practice, Training, 38, 4, pp. 345–356.

Norcross, J.C. and Lambert, M.J. [2018], *Psychotherapy relationships that work III*, in Psychotherapy, 55, 4, pp. 303–315.

Norcross, J.C. and Wampold, B.E. [2011], *What works for whom: tailoring psychotherapy to the person*, in Journal of Clinical Psychology, 67, pp. 127–132.

Oldham, J.M., Skodol, A.E., Kellman, H.D., Hyler, S.E., Doidge, N., Rosnick, L., *et al.* [1995], *Comorbidity of Axis I and Axis II disorders*, in American Journal of Psychiatry, 152, pp. 571–578.

Patterson, C.H. [1984], *Empathy, warmth, and genuineness in psychotherapy: a review of reviews*, in Psychotherapy: Theory, Research, Practice, Training, 21, 4, pp. 431–438.

Penn, P. and Frankfurt, M. [1994], *Creating a participant text: writing, multiple voices, narrative multiplicity*, in Family Process, 33, 3, pp. 217–231.

Prochaska, J.O. and Norcross, J.C. [2001], *Stages of change*, in Psychotherapy: Theory, Research, Practice, Training, 38, 4, pp. 443–448.

Rober, P. [2017], *In therapy together*, London, Palgrave.

Rosenzweig, S. [1936], *Some implicit common factors in diverse methods of psychotherapy*, in American Journal of Orthopsychiatry, 6, 3, pp. 412–415.

Roy-Chowdhury, S. [2006], *How is the therapeutic relationship talked into being?*, in Journal of Family Therapy, 28, 2, pp. 153–174.

Roy-Chowdhury, S. [2003], *Knowing the unknowable: what constitutes evidence in family therapy?*, in Journal of Family Therapy, 25, pp. 64–85.

Schegloff, E.A. [2007], *A primer in conversation analysis*, Cambridge MA, Cambridge University Press.

Seligman, M.E.P. [1995], *The effectiveness of psychotherapy*, in American Psychologist, 50, pp. 965–974.

Shotter, J. [1993], *Conversational realities*, London, Sage Publications.

Sprenkle, D.H. and Blow, A.J. [2004], *Common factors and our sacred models*, in Journal of Marital and Family Therapy, 30, 2, pp. 113–129.

Stratton, P., Bland, J., Janes, E. and Lask, J. [2010], *Developing an indicator of family function and a practicable outcome measure for systemic family and couple therapy: the SCORE*, in Journal of Family Therapy, 32, pp. 232–258.

Stiles, W.B., Barkham, M., Mellor-Clark, J. and Connell, J. [2008], *Effectiveness of cognitive-behavioural, person-centred, and psychodynamic therapies in UK primary-care routine practice: replication in a larger sample*, in Psychological medicine, 38, 5, pp. 677–688.

Swift, J.K., Callahan, J.L. and Vollmer, B.M. [2011], *Preferences*, in Journal of Clinical Psychology, 67, pp. 155–165.

Wampold, B.E. [2001], *The great psychotherapy debate: models, methods, and findings*, Mahwah, Lawrence Erlbaum Associates.

Wampold, B.E. [2015], *How important are the common factors in psychotherapy? An update*, in World Psychiatry, 14, 3, pp. 270–277.

Wampold, B.E. and Carlson, J. [2011], *Qualities and actions of effective therapists*, Washington DC, American Psychological Association.

Westen, D., Novotny, C.M. and Thompson-Brenner, H. [2004], *The empirical status of empirically supported psychotherapies: assumptions, findings, and reporting in controlled clinical trials*, in Psychological Bulletin, 130, 4, pp. 631–663.

Part I

Technical competency in systemic practice: the dialogical construction of a shared symbolic space

1 From diagnosis to care

The technical aspect of therapeutic competency refers to the knowledge of procedures, theories, and methods of intervention elaborated within a specific approach, and to the ability to translate them into practices that are expressions of such premises. In fact, every technical intervention is linked to a paradigm, a conceptual framework, which defines the practitioner's realm of investigation, conception of psychological problem, procedures to collect data, and methods of intervention. In our case, technical competency is linked to the systemic-constructionist paradigm.

The main assumption of the systemic approach is that it is neither possible to explain the development of individuls independently from their system (the network of relationships which they are part of), nor understand behaviours out of context (the circumstances and situations within which behaviours take place). In the past, the emphasis placed on family as a unit of analysis and intervention has driven to the development of methods that have influenced family therapy, thereby creating an overlap between systemic psychotherapy and family therapy. However, the epistemological, theoretical, and methodological development that has characterized systemic psychotherapy has gone beyond the exclusive identification with family therapy. Indeed, the systemic approach has rapidly proved to be a general model of analysis and intervention for therapies with individuals [Boscolo and Bertrando 1996; Hedges 2005], rehabilitation programmes [Castellucci, Fruggeri and Marzari 1985], integrated network therapies [Campbell and Draper 1985; Fruggeri et al. 1991], psycho-social interventions [McCarthy 1995], and psychological support programmes in healthcare services [Gritti 2015; Ruddy and McDaniel 2015].

The systemic perspective has transformed the ways in which symptoms, diagnoses, and treatments have been defined: these notions have been re-conceptualized in relational terms. More specifically, a symptom is not considered the expression of an individual dysfunction; rather, it is treated as information about the relational contexts of the client. Diagnosis is no longer conceived of as the attribution of pathological categories to an individual; rather, it refers to ways of group functioning. Lastly, the therapeutic intervention is based on the observation of patterns of interactions and dynamics of the whole family group, or in general, of the group to which the individual

DOI: 10.4324/9781003278092-3

belongs. Also, the intervention is aimed at changing the context within which the problem has emerged and has been maintained. In line with this paradigm, the systemic technical competency is the ability to observe from different points of view how individuals' behaviours can make sense within the relational dynamics of their families, or within the broader relational contexts they belong to, and use these "multiple views" to engage in conversations that can trigger change in clients' lives.

Methodological issues in psychotherapy

In the field of systemic psychotherapy, the issue of diagnosis has always been controversial.

The pioneers of family therapy were split between those who considered the diagnosis as a key tool for treatment [Ackerman 1958] and those who claimed it was not necessary [Haley 1970]. With the development of a rigorous epistemological reflection, an alternative paradigm for diagnosis based on cybernetics, ecology, and systems theory was proposed by several authors [Keeney 1979; Campbell *et al.* 1982]. The influence of social constructionism on the systemic approach has led to even more radical positions: diagnosis was considered dangerous. Several scholars have pointed out that the diagnostic categories, the language, and the heuristic principles used by therapists could contribute to the social construction of psychopathology, instead of contributing to the solution to the problem [Rosenhan 1973; Dell 1980; Watzlawick 1984; Anderson, Goolishian and Winderman 1986; Boscolo et al. 1987]. On a completely opposite position, others have proposed developing relational diagnostic categories to be included in the *Diagnostic and Statistical Manual of Mental Disorders* (DSM) alongside the individual categories [Klaslow 1993]. The use of the term "diagnosis" with different meanings has contributed to making this notion even more ambiguous. For these reasons, we are introducing some linguistic distinctions that can be helpful to differentiate the methodological tools according to coherence with their theoretical foundation and their function in the therapeutic process.

The term "diagnosis" refers to a procedure by which signs, or symptoms, are attributed to a predefined pathological category. In carrying out a diagnosis, practitioners search for clues that can lead them to discriminate between different clinical scenarios and eventually identify the correct one. The classic diagnostic categorization informed by a psychiatric approach is based on the premise that psychopathologies should be identified regardless of the observers and the theoretical framework they adopt. This approach is clearly expressed by the DSM [American Psychiatric Association 2013]. The DSM is one of the most popular psychopathological nosographic systems that define the various disorders using criteria universally shared and characterized as a-theoretical and functional. In this approach, the diagnostic process is an assessment based on the collection of data that allow clinicians to prepare for the intervention with the client. The psychiatric diagnostic approach has been subject to various criticisms in the psychotherapeutic field, namely the diagnostic categories describe psychological problems, not explain them; they tend to "biologize" psychological processes; and they contribute to hide personal and relational characteristics of individuals behind a label. Boscolo and colleagues [1987] stressed that once labelling has been accepted, then all behaviours are related to the labelling, and the psychiatric problem becomes the reference point to explain all behaviours of the designated patient.

In the process of distancing ourselves from psychiatric approaches to diagnosis, we are, however, introducing a different kind of map – one based on observation. Initiating a therapeutic encounter without observational categories places therapists at risk for unconsciously sharing the same vision and the same descriptive and interpretative categories of clients. This would prevent the therapists from bringing differences to the therapeutic conversation, whose effectiveness is based on letting emerge and identifying dissonances in clients' story [Cecchin 1987; Boscolo *et al.* 1987; Sluzki, 1992; Madonna 2003]. "Actively researching and enhancing the differences is a fundamental prerequisite for recognizing the client's potentials and resources for generating new knowledge useful to the therapeutic process" [Tramonti and Fanali 2013, p. 72]. To sustain clients' change and evolution, therapists should embrace divergent thinking and resist the tendency to seek stability and confirmation, as well as avoid explanations shared by common sense (see Chapter 6).

While refusing a psychiatric psychopathological classification, therapists will choose some methodological criteria to "make order" of the endless amount of information that every therapeutic encounter entails [Keeney 1983] and to maintain a curious stance toward clients: "When we feel unable to develop hypotheses, we know we have accepted the family's script, and thus, have lost our sense of curiosity" [Cecchin 1987, p. 411].

Paraphrasing Bateson [1972], all therapists will adopt a "map" that allows them to make sense of the information offered by clients about the "territory" of their story. In this sense, the central point of the discussion is what methodological criteria use and for what purpose. Methodological tools should be at the service of those who use them, that is, they should support practitioners in a functional and coherent way. In this sense, the nosological classification of psychopathologies is functional to psychiatrists who prescribe drugs, but it is useless to a systemic therapist who is interested in understanding the relational dynamics underlying the development of psychological distress and in listening to what clients consider as painful in their lives [Rober 2017]. Consider this case example.

Luis is 50 years old and lives with his parents: his mother is 78 years old, and his father is 82. Since he was a teenager, he has received assistance from the local mental health service. He currently has a job and lives a simple life with the support of his parents. This situation is disrupted when Luis's father develops dementia: the mother must take care of her husband; Luis becomes increasingly anxious, quits his work, and spends his days at home, arguing with his father. The situation becomes more and more difficult. The mother consults with the psychiatrists and makes clear that she cannot take care of two persons in need of constant help and assistance. The psychiatrists decide to transfer Luis to a residential rehabilitation centre where he can participate in different activities, be monitored from the pharmacological point of view, and spend time away from a stressful family context. The decision turns out to be good. Luis becomes gradually more active and takes part in the daily life routines of the community, such as helping with cleaning, setting the table, etc. At this point, the professionals of the residential centre estimate that it is time for him to pay a visit to his parents, so he does. However, once he is back at the residential centre, Luis seems to have regressed in several respects. He refuses to attend community activities and exhibits the following behaviour: he constantly checks his underpants or asks anyone he meets to do the same thing, to be reassured that he has not wet himself. The persistence of this symptom triggers a crisis in the community: nurses and doctors begin to think that Luis is "going crazy"; the other guests become annoyed and angry at Luis's behaviour. In other words, everyone in the community develops rejecting attitudes towards him. The professionals ask for a consultation with the supervisor in order to make sense of what they see as an incomprehensible regression, which they can only qualify in terms of pathology to the point of foreseeing Luis's admission to a psychiatric ward as the only solution. During the supervisory session, professionals are invited to report observations and explore ideas about what aspects could be linked to Luis's behaviour. Someone comments that his behaviour reminds them of a child who fears wetting himself. Someone else comments that this is a good idea, but where does this fear come from? The nurse who took Luis home said his mother was very happy to see him and showed great affection, and when she went to collect him to go back to the rehab centre, the mother said everything went very well. However, once in the car, Luis told the nurse that he had wanted to help his mother with cleaning, but his mother had said: "Don't worry; I'll do it when you are gone". Luis had offered to help, but his help was refused. The professionals link this episode to both Luis's symptom and the withdrawal from his job when his father started suffering from dementia. The team begins to identify a pattern: Luis had offered to help his mother, as an adult son would normally do, but his help had been systematically refused; in this sense, Luis has been treated as a little child. It is likely that the mother's intention was to protect Luis, not to belittle him, yet in Luis's experience, the mother's answer to his offer of help might have felt like an invalidation. This idea provided a possible line of interpretation for the symptom and allowed the team to develop a plan for a collaborative intervention focused on how Luis and his mother could help one another. The sessions with Luis and his mother revealed emotions, expectations, and possibilities, which paved the way to Luis's discharge from the rehab centre and to his return home.

This case example shows that the use of a diagnostic framework focused on psychopathology would have reified Luis's problem; instead, embracing a perspective focused on Luis's relational system and the meanings of his behaviour in that context allowed the team to become creative and develop a successful psychotherapeutic intervention based on collaboration. This type of intervention has transformed a diagnostic setting in a setting of care [Madonna 2003], namely a shared space for the emergence of a new language, new meanings, and new stories.

The systemic perspective sustains the idea that the therapist should understand things using different lenses. Practitioners should not position themselves outside the observed system, seeking what is not working in families or in clients' lives; they should rather act as participant observers, who contribute to construct clients' issues also through their point of view. In other words, practitioners as participant observers do not use static diagnostic categories (which can become labels for clients) but analyze the ongoing process they are part of. From this point of view, making sense of a problematic situation through giving meaning to what may appear senseless can be defined as an "… evolving assessment process recursively connected to the therapeutic effect of the therapist's investigation of one or more persons considered in their relational and emotional context" [Boscolo and Bertrando 1996, p. 51].

The systemic therapist cultivates the tension between understanding the dynamics connected to the problem and exploring possible solutions together with the clients. Understanding clients' worries and co-constructing with them new meanings that favour change are two inextricably interconnected processes; in fact, the same process of knowing is an inter-subjective activity that creates new meanings. This is an approach we define as *systemic*, since it focuses on contexts and relationships; *constructionist*, since it considers change as the outcome of an interactive process; and *dialogic*, because it stresses negotiation and collaboration among the participants in the process.

Hypothesizing as a dialogical process

Etymologically, hypothesis is defined as a supposition or proposed explanation based on limited evidence, as a starting point for further investigation (source: https://www.lexico.com/definition/hypothesis). Selvini Palazzoli and colleagues [1980] named *hypothesizing* as the therapists's ability to formulate a hypothesis based on the available information on the case and their knowledge to provide explanations of the problem brought by clients.

> The hypothesis establishes a starting point for his investigation as well as his verification of the validity of this hypothesis based upon specific methods and skills. If the hypothesis is proven false, the therapist must form a second hypothesis based upon the information gathered during the testing of the first.
>
> [Selvini Palazzoli *et al.* 1980, p. 3]

Despite the positivistic connotation of this definition, Selvini *et al.* underline that a hypothesis is neither true nor false, but helpful and functional to the development of conversations that introduce new points of view, differences, and connections among different pieces of information. Consistently, hypotheses should not be considered from the dichotomous perspective of confirming/disconfirming what is hypothesized, since the therapist does not seek general laws about systems' functioning. In fact, the therapist is part of a therapeutic relationship in which hypotheses coevolve with the family participation as the family's responses to the questioning modify or alter the previous hypothesis [Boscolo *et al.* 1987; Bertrando and Toffanetti 2000]. In this sense, the process of formulating hypotheses (in Selvini *et al.*'s terms: "hypothesizing"), should not be intended as a strategic way to guide clients toward a predetermined direction, thereby denying clients' subjectivity [Andersen 1991; Anderson and Goolishian 1992]; it should rather be considered as a way to make sense of psychopathological symptoms, which may appear senseless behaviours, and to foster conversations that create differences.

The formulation of hypotheses in a systemic framework was initially conceived as a "secret" plan of the therapist; however, over the years, it has been redefined in dialogical terms. Hypotheses are created, refined, changed, and shared with clients in the flow of therapeutic conversations: *both* therapists and clients participate in the systemic hypothesis formulation process [Bertrando and Arcelloni 2006]. Luis's case example, illustrated above, shows that hypotheses can serve the function of generating dialogues in which clients' subjectivity is included. Furthermore, it is worth noting that therapists observe and participate in systems that are not stable. In contrast to traditional diagnostic systems that provide a static image of clients' situations at a given time, systemic formulations allow therapists to acknowledge the dynamic nature of human systems since hypotheses develop and change according to clients' feedback.

Hypotheses can be considered "explicative schemas" [Ugazio 1985], that is, interpretations and attributions of meaning to one's own and to others' behaviours. Differently from schemas traditionally used in psychiatry or on the bases of "common sense", systemic hypotheses present some peculiarities. Firstly, they are at least triadic to introduce difference with respect to common sense dyadic or monadic interpretative explanations [Ugazio *et al.* 2012]. From a systemic point of view, the context of interactions is always triangular, since two interacting people are part of wider relational networks and each of them is involved in other significant relationships. Adopting a triadic approach to analyze the functioning of a group implies considering both the relationships and the contribution of each participant to that relationship, thereby addressing both relational and individual matters. Fruggeri [2018] stressed that the analysis of interactive processes in triadic contexts requires the use of the concept of *relational interdependence,* which describes mutual influences. According to the notion of relational interdependence, the meaning of the relationship between two people depends on the quality of the relationships that each of them has with significant others. A change in the quality or definition of the relationship brings changes to the quality or definition of the relationships that each of them has with others. In other words, a change in the dyadic relationship A-B reverberates on the dyadic relationship B-C, which reverberates on the dyadic relationship C-A [ibidem]. The concept of relational interdependence will be discussed in detail in Chapter 8.

Another peculiar aspect of systemic formulations is that hypotheses develop from information gathered at different logical levels. Inspiration for systemic explanations of specific situations can be found in the classic studies on communication and family dynamics [Wynne *et al.* 1958; Wynne 1961; Ferreira 1963; Satir 1964; Boszormenyi-Nagy and Framo 1965; Jackson 1965; Bowen 1966; Watzlawick, Beavin and Jackson 1967; Bateson 1972; Minuchin 1974; Selvini Palazzoli *et al.* 1978; Sluzki and Ramson 1976; Haley 1977] and in those subsequently elaborated [Selvini Palazzoli *et al.* 1989; Ugazio 2013], on models that have integrated the Theory of Attachment with family studies [Byng-Hall 1995; Dallos 2006] and others informed by a psychoanalytic approach applied to family relations [Wanlass and Scharff 2015]; as well as on many other contributions focusing on the cultural dimension of systems, on the developmental processes families undertake, and on other significant features characterizing family life [see Sexton and Lebov 2015]. However, the formulation of hypotheses relies on many more sources of information. First, the information contained in clients' idiosyncratic stories: systemic therapists consider clients as reliable sources of information regarding their feelings and experiences [Strong and Turner 2008]. Information collected for a clinical case is not only what clients narrate during the therapy session, but also all the pieces of information that therapists collect since the very first encounter with clients, such as: who contacted the therapists, whether clients have been referred and by whom, the urgency of the appointment, their tone of voice, etc. These pieces of information connect therapists to ideas, stories that will become objects of dialogue in the therapeutic encounter, which may or may not be accurate or useful [Hedges 2005]. Over the years, clinical practitioners develop an expertise based on schemes, analogies, metaphors, stories, and interventions, which can also be used to deal with new clinical cases [Fleuridas, Nelson and Rosenthal 1986]. Moreover, therapists' personality [Boscolo *et al.* 1987], their emotions emerging during the therapy session [Bertrando 2014; Lini and Bertrando 2020], their prejudices, and their heuristics contribute to hypotheses creation, too. Therefore, it is important for therapists to become aware of their premises and interpretations (see Chapters 5 and 6) to avoid becoming self-referential and losing the connection with clients' stories, feelings, and experiences.

Systemic hypothesising is an interactive and dynamic process since therapists' practice is guided by ideas that adapt and change according to clients' feedback. In this sense, hypothesising is a "stratification of provisional ideas" [Bertrando and Toffanetti 2000, 49]. The ability of therapists of changing hypotheses according to the interactive process they shape together with clients will be discussed in Chapter 4. Both therapists and clients are involved in a meaning-making process: therapists try to make sense of the problematic situation brought by the client, and explore, together with clients, different ways to connect the various elements of the system (relationships between people, meanings, stories, and points of view) with the aim of creating new and more useful patterns of meaning.

Asking (or not asking) a question, exploring (or not exploring) the problematic situation, and focusing on some information rather than on others can have different impacts on clients. The distinction between understanding and intervening is blurred: during therapeutic conversations, therapists and clients engage in a dialogue that potentially opens ways to consider the problem and its possible solutions that are new compared to those explored previously [Grossen 2006]. Strong [2011] has pointed out that therapist–client conversations are non-hierarchical in that the therapist dialogically values the client's contribution. Authors influenced by dialogism (see specifications in Box 1.1 below) emphasize the need for creating a space of expression for everyone involved, particularly giving voice to those marginalized and oppressed. Since systemic practice acknowledges and values clients' subjectivity, it can be conceived as a collaborative and co-evolutionary practice [McCarthy 2017]. It is in this framework that hypothesizing is considered here.

Box 1.1   Dialogism and dialogic practice by Federico Ferrari

Dialogism is a vision of the world based on respect for Otherness, listening, being with, and responding to the Other, to increase what Bakhtin [1984] calls "polyphony".

The "horizontal" polyphony is the coexistence, in the conversation, of several voices or points of view, distinct and equally valid. Promoting horizontal polyphony means: 1) creating space for each voice, bringing out the voices of those who remain silent, more hesitant, disoriented, or difficult to understand, and reducing the distance between those who are considered "ill" and those who are "healthy" [Olson, Seikkula and Ziedonis 2014]; and 2) encouraging a reflective process whereby the different voices do not just "coexist" but resonate and reflect on each other.

The "vertical" polyphony is the coexistence, in the internal dialogue of each person, of different voices that "arise" according to the themes of the dialogue and the person's resonances. Promoting vertical polyphony means accepting ambivalences and inner conflicts related to the possibility of different positions in the relationship. This is true for patients and therapists. The latter, for example, participate in the dialogue with the voices of their scientific competency, with those of their clinical methodology and their relational competency, but also with their personal and intimate voices [Seikkula 2008]. Dialogue and polyphony increase when "monological discourse" decreases. Monological discourse is a way of speaking in which the individual, as a privileged expert, speaks from top to bottom, without the contribution of the listener, thus hindering a collaborative process.

As a psychotherapeutic practice, dialogism is based on 2 basic skills: 1) responding, that is, making the other feel heard, understood, and recognized in the conversation; and 2) reflecting, that is, engaging in an open, participatory, transparent, and non-technical conversation.

Olson, Seikkula and Ziedonis [2014] identify 12 key conversational elements that generate and promote the flow of dialogue for the therapist:

1 Having 2 or more therapists present during the meeting;
2 Having the participation of the family and the network;
3 Using open-ended questions;
4 Always answering (even non-verbally) the patients' utterances;
5 Focusing on the present moment;
6 Stimulating multiple points of view;
7 Maintaining a relational lens in the dialogue;
8 Responding by paying attention to the concrete implications of problems and their meaning to people;
9 Emphasizing clients' words and stories, not their symptoms;
10 Conversing (reflecting) between professionals during the meeting;
11 Being transparent about one's own internal voices; and
12 Tolerating uncertainty.

Hypotheses "in action"

As discussed earlier, systemic practice frames therapist–client relationship as non-hierarchical. However, therapists continue to hold responsibility for including aspects of difference and dissonance into the therapeutic dialogue.

When clients, families, or couples decide to start psychotherapy, they bring a structured story and rigid explanations of the problem; the therapist tries to make them more flexible:

> Families are wonderful story tellers because they have such interesting scripts to describe. They come to therapy with these scripts tightly written. Their problem is that their scripts do not help them function in a way that they find useful. As clinicians, we offer the family new scripts (based on our hypotheses) to which the family responds by adjusting its script that, in turn, helps us alter our scripts, and so on.
> [Cecchin 1987, p. 411]

The continuous exchanges between the story of the client and the "story" of the therapist make hypothesis formulation a continuous co-evolutionary process [Boscolo *et al.* 1987]. In fact, hypothesizing builds upon the principle of circularity [Selvini Palazzoli *et al.* 1980], which refers to the ability to conduct conversations based on clients' (individual, couple, family) feedback to the information solicited by the therapist in terms of relationships, thus difference and change. Focusing on clients' feedback means that the therapist should be ready to face unexpected situations. In other words, therapists should capture everything happening in the therapeutic encounter and "reflect while acting" to adapt their responses to clients' feedback, modifying the intervention and the working hypothesis as well. Karl Tomm [1987] used the notion of *strategizing* to describe an intentional process through which therapists plan their actions to achieve a therapeutic goal. Strategizing is a conceptual stance (a set of operations aimed at supporting thoughts and actions) that allows therapists to reflect upon both the criteria for conducting the session and the verbal actions to be used during a therapeutic conversation. During psychotherapy sessions, therapists have the common experience of wondering about questions such as: "How could I explore this aspect? Whom should I ask this question to? What effect may have if I ask this question now? What's the meaning of talking about this now?" and so on.

In a more or less conscious way, in therapeutic sessions therapists are constantly wondering about their positioning. This aspect has been explored by Rober [2005; 2011] through the concept of *inner dialogue*, which is based on the dialogical premise that the speaker mentally anticipates the interlocutor's answer. When therapists listen to the stories of families, they not only "record" families' words, but these same words also resonate within them, stimulating an internal dialogue. Based on this dialogue, therapists respond to clients, who, in turn, develop conversations in relation to the inner dialogue triggered by therapists' words.

Gail Simon [2016, p. 171] has defined systemic practice as a form of research that emerges as a transformative practice since the process of inquiry leads to change and newness. As she writes: "We [systemic therapists] are listening for information and reflecting on what we think we have heard. We check on our first understanding – and our second, and our third … we ask what makes a difference … we look out for feedback … we invite other perspectives … we attend to internal and external dialogues. We make meaning and offer accounts. We review our theories".

Consider this case example.

The therapist is contacted by a man who would like to start psychotherapy. George, 38 years old (accountant), contacts the practitioner for a problem that has started about 6 months earlier: outbursts of anger, severe headaches, and insomnia. He consulted his general practitioner, who carried out some health checks and then referred him to a psychotherapist. He has been married for 7 years. His wife, Molly, is 36 years old, and they have a 4-year-old son. In the first interview, George tells the therapist that his current problem relates to his relationship with his in-laws (John and Mary, both 62 years old and retired). In particular, he has problems with his mother-in-law, described as an extremely intrusive, snooty, and pedantic person. George claims he has tried to understand her and to get along with her without success. He feels overwhelmed and jittery to the extent that he cannot sleep at night. When he got married, his in-laws offered for the couple to live in a small apartment in the same building: George says he was happy with that, and things have gone well for some years. Mary (the mother-in law) has always supported the daughter and George with childcare; however, she always wants the last word. A year earlier, George and his wife decided to look for a new house because they needed more space; they found an apartment near the in-laws' house, where they moved 6 months ago. George saw this change as a possible solution to the problem; however, he realized that nothing has changed. John and Mary questioned George and Molly's choice to leave their building; George feels hurt more than ever.

Starting from this information, the therapist begins to reflect upon this situation and decides to ask a question to identify the effects of George's problem:

Therapist: In what ways and in what moments has your problem had an impact on your everyday life?

George: It has a big impact … especially in the evening and weekends. At work it is fine, it is tiring from time to time, but overall, I am happy with my job. Actually, my job helps me not to think of the problems I have. Sometimes I can hardly sleep. In that case, it's difficult to work, but once I'm there, I am fine. Instead, once I'm back home, problems also come back. It's hard … especially during weekends.

At this point, the therapist wonders whom this man is close to and whom he can talk with; therefore, she asks the following question:

Therapist: Who is worried about your problem?

George: Well, my wife … she worries a lot! Over the last months, she has been very close to me, especially when I get severe migraines. She came with me to see a specialist, and she insisted that I do some health checks to make sure there is nothing to worry about such as cancer or an aneurysm.

Since George has mentioned his wife, the therapist decides to further explore this aspect. In fact, the investigation of the client's relational context in individual sessions has been shown to be of significant therapeutic value [Athanasiades 2008]:

Therapist: What does your wife think about this situation?

George: My wife is very sorry for me, especially because I am physically sick. But she barely understands the problems with my mother-in-law.

Therapist: What is it that your wife does not understand?

George: Molly does not understand that her mother's behaviour and attitude are totally wrong! She ignores that ... instead, I expect her to explain to her mother what is actually going on. For instance, the issue of the house ... my in-laws think we moved because I did not want to stay there; they told me: "we are not bad people".

The therapist wants to know more about the relationship between George's wife and her mother, thus enlarging the context to a triadic one:

Therapist: George, I am wondering how you would describe the relationship between your wife and your mother-in-law?
George: Molly relies on her mother's help for everything, especially for what concerns our child. When she has a problem, a wonder, a doubt, she calls her mother. You know, she is the only child ... she is terribly close to her mother.

The therapist has collected enough information to formulate a hypothesis, namely a provisional plausible explanation of George's problem. The therapist hypothesizes that George is suffering from the current situation, and in particular, from the relationship with the mother-in-law, because he feels his wife does not legitimize his role as a father. In fact, George stressed that his wife relies on her mother "for everything", including their child's care and education. To explore further this hypothesis, the therapist decides to ask the following questions:

Therapist: If your wife relied on you instead of her mother when she needs help, how do you think you would feel?
George: Well, I don't know ... it never happens ... but I think I would be happy. I mean, if she would consider my opinions and my ideas, I would feel recognized.
Therapist: In your view, do you think that your mother-in-law would change her behaviour, if you and your wife worked as a team when caring for your child and dealing with other issues of your family?
George: Well ... yes, it may be. She might stop intruding in our life.

George's answers regarding both the idea that he could feel better and that the mother-in-law would become less intrusive allow the therapist to proceed with further explorations in that direction.

This case illustrates that hypotheses orient the therapist's approach and actions, allowing for the selection of one question rather than another. This happens through a process that is not unidirectional, but it emerges from the interaction with clients: clients' answers to therapists' questions trigger therapists' connection to their internal dialogue, and recursively to their hypotheses, which can be confirmed, redefined, expanded, or even discarded. In this sense, the technical competence of a systemic therapist is mainly a dialogical competence. The literature provides several resources helpful to guide therapists to develop therapeutic conversations that can be generative of new meanings. In the next chapter, we will introduce the techniques that can guide and promote therapeutic conversations that are collaborative and co-generative of change.

Hypothesizing and therapists' positioning

As Burnham and Harris [2002] have pointed out, the process of hypothesizing can also be seen as part of the process of being transparent about the practitioners' ideas and cultural values so that they can be available for analysis and eventually for change.

Since the Feminist Studies of the 1980s and the socio-cultural analysis of psychotherapy that followed [Hare-Mustin 1978; McGoldrick, Anderson and Walsh 1989; Walters 1990], a new awareness has developed among systemic therapists due to the acknowledgement that psychotherapists and service users come from different cultures or have different social status, and as such, they meet in the therapeutic encounter bringing in different perspectives. But not only that: the differences that may characterize the protagonists of the therapeutic process (clients and therapists) are socially defined and hierarchically ordered, thus connoting their relationships in terms of power. In this sense, practice and systemic theory is not neutral but infused with cultural biases.

These considerations deeply influenced the process of hypothesizing in various ways, all concerning the therapists' position in it.

First, when making sense of the clients' difficulties and worries, therapists should consider how differences in gender, power, social, cultural, and economic conditions can affect personal conditions and the organization of interpersonal relationships.

Second, while hypothesizing therapists cannot avoid considering their participation in the process and looking out for the biases embedded in their social position.

Third, a reflection is needed about how power plays out in the therapeutic relationship; that is how the position of therapist might silence the voices of minorities and members of oppressed communities.

Fourth, therapists should be aware that if guided by models that ignore the differences created by social relations, they can inadvertently and unconsciously help to reconstruct these differences, as well as perpetuate the oppression and discrimination that such differences entail [James and McIntyre 1983]. For example, the therapists' ignorance of how gender stereotypes construct the inequality of power between males and females in families, helps to validate the conditions of this inequality [Goldner 1985; Lannamann 1991]; neglecting how poverty can contribute to triggering dysfunctional family dynamics, puts the therapist in a position to participate in the process of reproducing social inequalities [Jones 1994; McCarthy 1995]; limiting oneself, in therapy with gay and lesbian couples, to dealing with intra-family problems, without turning attention to how the tensions deriving from social discrimination towards this group of people can affect these problems, contributes to perpetuating their stigmatization [Bepko and Johnson 2000]; underestimating how much the ethnicity of families defines both their power relations at the social level and their interpersonal relationships, in fact corresponds to an assimilationist attitude that leaves minority cultures the only option to adapt to the dominant one [Falicov 1995].

> A lack of awareness of the wider political contexts which shape cross-cultural encounters, an insistence that benign intentions count for more than they do, an inability to reach into the complexity of institutional racism can, because of their subtlety, be as oppressive as some of the more obvious manifestation of racist practice.
>
> [Daniel 2012, pp. 93–94]

Social awareness leads family therapists to reflect on how much their interventions might unconsciously contribute to perpetuating the negative judgement on family forms different from the traditional ones and thus keeping them in the area of pathology or deviance.

These aspects of the process of hypothesizing gain particular relevance in supervision and training programs where therapists are educated to become aware of the ethical stances implied in psychotherapy: the choice between reinforcing dominant colonizing norms or contributing to overcome them through decolonizing practices [see for example Burnham and Harris 2002; Sing and Chun 2010; Pendry 2012; Burnham 2012; Reynolds and Larcombe 2016].

We will discuss these issues further in Part III and IV of the book.

References

Ackerman, N. [1958], *The psychodynamics of family life*, New York, Basic Books.

American Psychiatric Association [2013], *DSM-5. Diagnostic and Statistical Manual of Mental Disorders*.

Athanasiades, C. [2008], *Systemic thinking and circular questioning in therapy with individuals*, in Counselling Psychology Review, 23, 3, pp. 5–13.

Andersen, T. [1991], *The reflecting team: dialogues and dialogues about the dialogues*, New York, W.W. Norton & Co.

Anderson, H. and Goolishian, H. [1992], *The client is the expert: a not-knowing approach to therapy*, in S. McNamee and K.J. Gergen (eds), *Inquiries in social construction. Therapy as social construction*, London, Sage, pp. 25–39.

Anderson, H., Goolishian, H. and Winderman, L. [1986], *Problem determined systems: toward a transformation in family therapy*, in Journal of Strategic and Systemic Therapies, 5, pp. 14–19.

Bachtin, M. [1984], *Problems of dostoevsky' poetics*. Minneapolis, University of Minnesota Press.

Bateson, G. [1972], *Steps to an ecology of mind*, New York, Chandler.

Bepko, C. and Johnson, T. [2000], *Gay and lesbian couples in therapy: perspectives for the contemporary family therapist*, in Journal of Marital and Family Therapy, 26, pp. 409–419.

Bertrando, P. [2014], *Emotions and the therapist*, London, Karnac Books.

Bertrando, P., and Arcelloni, T. [2006], *Hypotheses are dialogues: sharing hypotheses with clients*, in Journal of Family Therapy, *28*, 4, pp. 370–387.

Bertrando, P. and Toffanetti, D. [2000], *Sull'ipotesi. Teoria e clinica del processo di ipotizzazione*, in Terapia Familiare, 62, pp. 43–68.

Boscolo, L. and Bertrando, P. [1996], *Systemic therapy with individuals*, London, Routledge.

Boscolo, L., Cecchin, G., Hoffman, L. and Penn, P. [1987], *Milan systemic family therapy*, New York, Basic Books.

Boszormenyi-Nagy, I. and Framo, J. (eds.) [1965], *Intensive family therapy*, New York, Harper and Row.

Bowen, M. [1966], *The use of family theory in clinical practice*, in Comprehensive Psychiatry, 7, 5, pp. 345–374.

Burnham, J. [2012], *Developments in Social GRRRAAACCEEESSS: visible–invisible and voiced–unvoiced*, in B. Kruse (ed), *Culture and reflexivity in systemic psychotherapy*, London, Karnac, pp. 139 -160.

Burnham, J. and Harris, Q. [2002], *Cultural issues in supervision*, in, D. Campbell and B. Mason (eds), *Perspectives in supervision*, London, Karnak, pp. 21–41

Byng-Hall, J. [1995], *Re-writing family scripts*, New York, Guilford Press.

Campbell, D.E., Steenbarger, B.N., Smith, T.W. and Stucky, R.J. [1982], *An ecological systems approach to evaluation: cruising in topeka*, in Evaluation review, 5, pp. 625–648.

Campbell, D. and Draper, R. (eds) [1985], *Applications of systemic family therapy: the Milan Method*, London, Grune and Stratton.

Castellucci, A., Fruggeri, L. and Marzari, M. [1985], *Instability and evolutionary change in a psychiatric community*, in D. Campbell and R. Draper (eds.), *Applications of systemic family therapy: the Milan Method*, London, Grune and Stratton, pp. 181–189.

Cecchin, G. [1987], *Hypothesizing, circularity, and neutrality revisited: an invitation to curiosity*, in Family Process, 26, 4, pp. 405–413.

Dallos, R. [2006], *Attachment narrative therapy*, New York, McGraw Hill.

Daniel, G. [2012], *With an exile's eye: developing positions of cultural reflexivity (with a bit of help from feminism)*, in B. Krause (ed.) *Culture and reflexivity in systemic psychotherapy*, London, Karnac, pp. 91–113.

Dell, P. [1980], *Researching the family theories of schizophrenia: an exercise in epistemological confusion*, in Family Process, 19, pp. 321- 335.

Falicov, C.J. [1995], *Training to think culturally: a multidimensional comparative perspective*, in Family Process, 34, pp. 373–388.

Ferreira, A. [1963], *Family myths and homeostasis*, in Archives of General Psychiatry, n. 9, pp. 457–463.

Fleuridas, C., Nelson, T. and Rosenthal, D. [1986], *The evolution of circular questions: training family therapists*, in Journal of Marital and Family Therapy, 12, 2, pp. 113–127.

Fruggeri, L. (ed.) [2018], *Famiglie d'oggi: quotidianità, dinamiche e processi psicosociali*, Roma, Carocci.

Fruggeri, L., Telfener, U., Castellucci, A., Marzari, M. and Matteini, M. [1991], *New systemic ideas from the Italian mental health movement*, London, Karnac Books.

Goldner, V. [1985], *Feminism and family therapy*, in Family Process, 24, pp. 31–47.

Gritti, P. [2015], *Family meetings in oncology: some practical guidelines*, in Frontiers in Psychology, 5, pp. 1552.

Grossen, M. [2006], *Analyse de la demande et construction du «problème» dans un premier entretien clinique*, in M. Grossen eA. Salazar Orvig, (eds.), *L'entretien clinique en pratiques*, Paris, Belin, pp.129–147.

Haley, J. [1970], *Possible approaches to family therapy*, in International Journal of Psychiatry, 9, pp. 233–242.

Haley, J. [1977], *Toward a theory of pathological systems*, in P. Watzlawick and J. Weakland (eds.), *The interactional view*, New York, Norton.

Hare Mustin, R. [1978], *A feminist approach to family therapy*, in Family Process, 17, pp. 181–194.

Hedges, F. [2005], *An introduction to systemic therapy with individuals. A social constructionist approach*, London, Palgrave Macmillan.

Jackson, D.D. [1965], *The study of the family*, in Family Process, 4, pp. 1–20.

James, K. and McIntyre, D. [1983], *The reproduction of families*, in Journal of Marital and Family Therapy, 9, pp. 119–129.

Jones, E. [1994], *Gender and poverty: a context for depression*, in Human Systems, 5, pp. 169–183.

Keeney, B.P. [1979], *Ecosystemic epistemology: an alternative paradigm for diagnosis*, in Family Process, 18, 2, pp. 117–129.

Keeney, B.P. [1983], *Aesthetics of change*, New York, Guilford Press.

Klaslow, F.W. [1993], *Relational diagnosis: an idea whose time has come?*, in Family Process, 32, 2, pp. 255–259.

Lannamann, J. [1991], *Interpersonal communication. Research and ideological practice*, in Communication Theory, 1991, 31, pp. 179–203.

Lini, C. and Bertrando, P. [2020], *Finding one's place: emotions and positioning in systemic-dialogical therapy*, in Journal of Family Therapy, 42, 2, pp. 204–221.

Madonna, G. [2003], *La psicoterapia attraverso Bateson*, Milano, Franco Angeli.

McCarthy, I. (ed.) [1995], *Irish family studies: selected papers*, UCD, Family Studies Center.

McCarthy, I. [2017], *The ocean in the waves: unity in diversity and the implications of a Fifth Province approach in complex systems*, in Metalogos Systemic Therapy Journal, 31.

McGoldrick, M., Anderson, C. and Walsh, F. [1989], *Women in families*. New York, Norton.

Minuchin, S. [1974], *Families and family therapy*, Cambridge, MA, Harvard University Press.

Olson, M., Seikkula, J. and Ziedonis, D. [2014], *The key elements of dialogic practice in open dialogue: fidelity criteria*, Worcester MA, The University of Massachusetts Medical School.

Pendry, N. [2012], *Race, racism and systemic supervision*, in Journal of Family Therapy, 34, pp. 403–418.

Reynolds, V. and Larcombe, A. [2016], *Living supervision in practice*, in I. McCarthy and G. Simon (eds.), *Systemic therapy as transformative practice*, Farnhill, UK, Everything is Connected Press, pp. 125–138.

Rober, P. [2005], *Family therapy as a dialogue of living persons*, in Journal of Marital and Family Therapy, 31, pp. 385–397.

Rober, P. [2011], *The therapists experiencing in family therapy*, in Journal of Marital and Family Therapy, 33, pp. 233–255.

Rober, P. [2017], *In therapy together*, London, Palgrave.

Rosenhan, D. [1973], *On being sane in insane places*, in Science, 179, pp. 250–258.

Ruddy, N. and McDaniel S.H. [2015], *Medical family therapy*, in T.L. Sexton and J. Lebow (eds.), *Handbook of family therapy*, New York, Routledge, pp. 471–484.

Satir, V. [1964], *Conjoint family therapy*, Palo Alto CA, Science and Behavior Books.

Seikkula, J. [2008], *Inner and outer voices in the present moment of family and network therapy*, in Journal of Family Therapy, 30, 4, pp. 478–491.

Selvini Palazzoli, M., Boscolo, L., Cecchin, G. and Prata, G. [1978], *Paradox and counter-paradox: a new model in the therapy of the family in schizophrenic transaction*, Northvale NJ, United States, Jason Aronson.

Selvini Palazzoli, M., Boscolo, L., Cecchin, G. and Prata, G. [1980], *Hypothesizing-circularity-neutrality: three guidelines for the conduction of session*, in Family Process, 19, 1, pp. 3–12.

Selvini Palazzoli, M., Cirillo, S., Selvini, M. and Sorrentino, A.M. [1989], *Family games: general models of psychotic processes in the family*, Hardcover, W.W. Norton & Company.

Sexton T.L. and Lebow J. (eds.) [2015], *Handbook of family therapy. The science and practice of working with families and couples*, New York, Routledge.

Simon, G. [2016] *Systemic practice as systemic inquiry as transformative research*, in I. McCarthy and G. Simon, (eds), *Systemic therapy as transformative practice*, Farnhill (UK), Everything is Connected Press, pp. 169–191.

Sing, A. and Chun, K.Y. [2010], *From the margin to the center: moving toward a resilience. Based model of supervision for queer people of color supervisors*, in Training and education in professional Psychology, 4, p. 36–46.

Sluzki, C. [1992], *Transformations: a blueprint for narrative changes in therapy*, in Family Process, 31, pp. 217–230.

Sluzki, C. and Ramson, D. [1976], *Double bind*, New York, Grune and Stratton.

Strong, T. [2011], *Flattening hierarchies? Thoughts on collaboration and psychological dialogues that clients might consider socially just*, in International Journal for Dialogical Science, 5, 1, pp. 1–16.

Strong, T. and Turner, K. [2008], *Resourceful dialogues: eliciting and mobilizing client competencies and resources*, in Journal of Contemporary Psychotherapy, 38, pp. 185–195

Tomm, K. [1987], *Interventive interviewing, part I: strategizing as a fourth guideline for the therapist*, in Family Process, 26, pp. 3–13.

Tramonti, F. and Fanali, A. [2013], *Identità e legami. La psicoterapia individuale a indirizzo sistemico-relazionale*, Firenze, Giunti.

Ugazio, V. [1985], *Hypothesis making*, in C. Campbell and R. Draper (eds), *Application of Systemic Family Therapy*, London, Grune and Stratton, pp. 23–32.

Ugazio, V. [2013], *Semantic polarities and psychopathologies in the family: permitted and forbidden stories*, London, Routledge.

Ugazio, V., Fellin, L., Pennacchio, R., Negri, A. and Colciago, F. [2012], *Is systemic thinking extraneous to common sense?* in Journal of Family Therapy, 34, pp. 53–71.

Walters M. [1990], *A feminist perspective in family therapy*, in R.J. Perelberg, A.C. Miller (eds), *Gender and power in families*, London, Routledge, pp. 13–33.

Wanlass, J. and Scharff D.E. [2015], *Psychodynamic approaches to couple and family therapy*, in T.L. Sexton and J. Lebow (eds.), *Handbook of family therapy*, New York, Routledge, pp. 120–145.

Watzlawick, P. (ed.) [1984], *The invented reality*, New York, Norton.

Watzlawick, P., Beavin, J.H. and Jackson, D.D. [1967], *Pragmatics of human communication*. New York, W.W. Norton & Co.

Wynne, L. [1961], *The study of intrafamilial alignments and splits in exploratory family therapy*, in N.W. Ackerman, F. Beatman and S.N. Sherman (eds.), *Exploring the base for family therapy*, New York, Family Service Association of America, pp. 95–115.

Wynne, L., Ryckoff, I.M., Day, J. and Hirish S. [1958], *Pseudomutuality in the family relations of schizophrenics*, in Psychiatry, 21, pp. 205–220.

2 Technical support for dialogical competency

Hypothesizing is a dynamic process that takes place in the conversational exchange between the therapist and clients, in which practitioners' interventions, based on the available techniques, contribute to generating new information useful to the process itself.

Over time, several authors have developed and described techniques for conducting the session [Penn 1982; 1985; Fleuridas, Nelson and Rosenthal 1986; Tomm 1987a; 1987b; 1988; McCarthy and Byrne 1988; Brown 1997; Byrne and McCarthy 2007; among others]. Questions are the main tool of the systemic therapist: in line with the theoretical approach, they are based on hypotheses, which in turn are elaborated by connecting ideas, narratives, emotions, experiences, and premises.

As pointed out, hypothesizing is a continuously evolving process: it develops in conversation, and it is through questions that therapists propose their hypothesis, and consistently with the feedback they receive from the client(s), enlarge or modify it. Questions are an effective tool for knowledge, discovery, and change. Learning how to formulate questions supports dialogical ability, and knowing how to ask questions is an art that can be taught.

Questions aim to widen the points of view on the story that is presented. They do not take the form of statements, advice, or prescriptions, but rather propose an open reflection. The interlocutory structure of questions leaves freedom to clients; it prevents them from proceeding alone – thus ending up telling the same story over and over again. Questions collect and give information. They have both an exploratory and a transformative function.

In this chapter, some classifications of questions that are accessible in the literature will be described. They constitute a set of tools available to therapists and are meant to be used within the complex theoretical and methodological framework described in the previous chapters. The set of questions proposed here do not cover the immense literature on this subject; it is a selection that we consider interesting, because it illustrates various types of questions that may have different functions in the conversation. Questions can: foster the exploration of the situation; stimulate clients' reflexivity; help clients to decentre; consider the existence of different points of view; encourage a multiple understanding of events, behaviours, and feelings; connect different

DOI: 10.4324/9781003278092-4

information; and help clients to tell their own story by introducing new elements. In this sense, questions are a technical support for the development of psychotherapists' dialogical competency. While each question has its own specificity, they all have the common goal of nurturing a transformative dialogue.

The question cube

Edward Brown [1997] identified specific elements that contribute to the formulation of a question. When combined, these elements give shape to a multiplicity of different interventions, each with its own dialogic function. In particular, the author outlines a 3-dimensional model that breaks questions into 3 components: *format*, which refers to the style of the question (open, closed, forced choice, rating, or ranking); *orientation*, which can be towards oneself or towards others; and *subject*, which classifies questions in terms of content or context. All these components and their respective levels can be combined to form different types of questions with specific functions (see Figure 2.1).

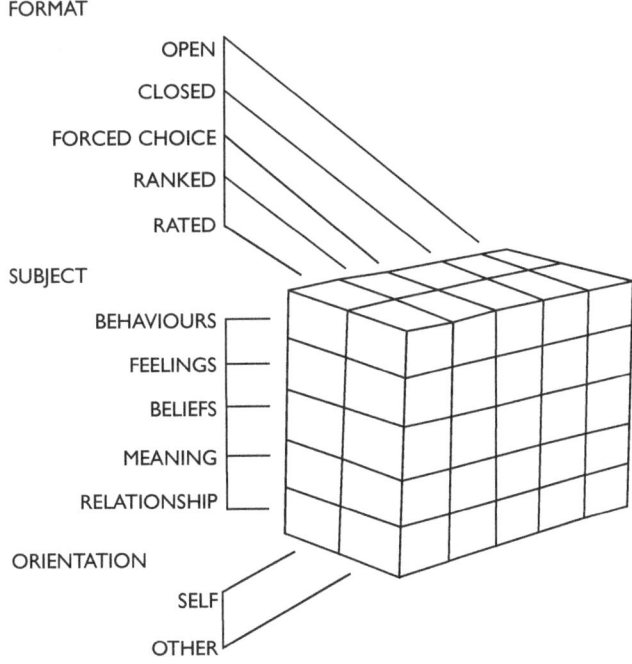

Figure 2.1 The question cube [Brown 1997].

The format of the questions

The format refers to the question's degree of openness. The more structured the question, the less information is required from the client. From this point of view, 5 types of questions can be identified:

⇒ *Open questions* offer greater freedom of response to clients while allowing the therapist to obtain more information. When clients tend to answer with just 1 word, this type of question can help them to further elaborate their response. Examples are as follows: *How would you describe your relationship with your sister? What do your parents think of your career?*

⇒ *Closed questions* are the most structured; they lead to short answers and are useful for obtaining specific information. These questions are often discouraged in therapy precisely because of the brevity of the answers they prompt; however, if the right question is asked at the right time, even a brief response can be meaningful. Closed questions are particularly useful when the therapist looks for a quick and relevant answer. Examples are as follows: *Do you get on well with your work colleagues? Do you think your parents were disappointed by your choice to withdraw from university?*

⇒ *Forced choice questions* are also highly structured, as they require the client to answer by choosing one of the options presented. When a client is having difficulties with an open question, a forced-choice question with 2 or more alternatives can make the response easier. These questions can have the function of making equally acceptable different answers and can provide insights that allow clients to think about their situation in a new way. Examples are as follows: *Do you think your relationship with your partner was better before you had your daughter because you talked to each other more or because you both had interesting jobs? "Does your family think that you should come to therapy as a way of helping you put up with a difficult situation or as a way to help you change the situation?"* [Brown 1997, p. 30].

⇒ *Ranking questions* require clients to classify family members on behaviours, feelings, and beliefs or understanding of particular events and relationships. Ranking questions are a subtle way of communicating to clients that some characteristics concern not just 1 person but are to some extent distributed among all family members. For example, if a family member is described as absent-minded, a ranking question might ask: *Who is the most absent-minded? Who is next most inattentive? Who is the least inattentive in the family?* Classification questions are also useful to investigate the emotional climate of the family in relation to the presented issue: *"If you were answering for your partner, who in the family would he say is most concerned about the problem of managing your children's behaviour? Who next?"* [Brown 1997, p. 31]. *If you look back to a year ago when you found out that your child was not going to school, who do you think was more surprised? Who next?*

⇒ *Rating questions* are aimed at assessing specific behaviours, beliefs, feelings, attitudes, situations, or relationships by asking clients to rate them on a scale of

1 to 10. Questions of this type can be addressed to each family member to compare different points of view. Rating questions can be a further refinement of ranking questions when a more focused view is required. Examples are as follows: *How satisfied are you with your relationship on a scale of 1 (very dissatisfied) to 10 (extremely satisfied)? How would you rate your degree of distress regarding the situation you are experiencing on a scale from 1 to 10?*

The orientation of the questions

Orientation indicates to whom the questions refer. Questions can ask something about oneself or about others.

⇒ *Self-oriented questions* are asked to explore clients' self-perceptions about their own thoughts, feelings, behaviour, and motivations. This type of question is among the most common and is widely used in all types of interviews. Examples are as follows: *What did you do when your partner told you she was in another relationship? What do you think of your current situation?*

⇒ *Other-oriented questions* are useful for exploring perceptions of another person's behaviour, feelings, motives, and beliefs. These questions foster the idea that there is more than 1 point of view on any given situation. Examples are as follows: *"Do you think your partner was angrier or sadder when you told him you were leaving him?" "How do you think that your parents would describe their relationship?"* [Brown 1997, p. 33].

The subject of the questions

The subject of a question concerns the type of information that is asked and may refer to *content* or *context*.

⇒ *Content* questions are intended to obtain basic information about the client's situation and may relate to behaviours, feelings, and beliefs.

Questions about *behaviours* are usually the first to be asked. These are the questions that clients are most likely to answer, as they tend to be more familiar with talking about behaviours than feelings or beliefs. Examples are as follows: *"What did your partner do when s/he found out that s/he had lost her/his job?"* [Brown 1997, p. 34]. *What did you do when your mother scolded you?*

Questions about *feelings* help to paint a more vivid picture of the motivation for a behaviour and its impact on others. These kinds of questions allow understanding that certain behaviours can evoke different feelings and therefore play a central role in understanding clients' perceptions and meanings. They also help to increase empathy between family members, as knowing feelings helps to interpret behaviour. Examples are as follows: *"Does your brother feel more love or hate for your father right now?"* [Brown 1997, p. 35]. *How did you feel when you found out that your friend was seriously ill?*

The purpose of *belief* questions is to try to understand the origin of certain ways of behaving, feeling, or thinking. These questions are particularly useful when exploring topics such as family of origin, culture, religion, social class, gender, sexual preference, and commonly shared social opinions. Examples are as follows: *"What beliefs about remaining with your partner through thick and thin did you bring with you from your family of origin?"* [Brown 1997, p. 35]. *Where do you think your wife got the idea of not being allowed to show sadness in front of your children?*

⇒ *Context* questions are proposed to reflect on the information obtained. They are meta-questions and refer to the general meaning attributed by clients to the content or to the type of relationship that emerges from the content.

Questions about *meanings* help clients to decentre understanding how their behaviour can be interpreted by others, and to comprehend the responses that their behaviour elicits. Examples are as follows: *"When you stayed out all night the evening you lost your job, what message were you trying to convey to your partner?"* [Brown 1997, p. 35]. *Who believes most that you should leave your partner?*

Relationship questions are used to highlight how behaviour is related to the nature of the relationship. Answering these questions allows clients to reflect on the impact of behaviours, feelings, and beliefs on their relationships. Examples are as follows: *"When he is sad and his mother comforts him, does that bring them closer together because they understand each other better or because they are afraid that the sadness will create an even greater rift?"* [Brown 1997, p. 36]; *How would you rate your commitment to rebuilding the relationship with your brother on a scale of 1 to 10?*

From a didactic point of view, this model suggests exploring all the components of the cube, practicing questions characterized by different combinations, and reflecting on the possible different effects that each combination can produce. As Brown [1997] points out, this model adds to therapists' toolbox a wealth of questions useful for the hypothesizing process.

Lineal, circular, strategic, and reflexive questions

Karl Tomm is one of the earliest and most important scholars in the field of therapeutic questioning [Boscolo and Bertrando 1996]. His work has been most widely disseminated in the family and couple therapy field. Tomm examined in depth the interview process that develops during a session and considered the whole interview as a series of continuous interventions. As he states, "everything an interviewer does and says, and does not do and does not say, is thought of as an intervention that could be therapeutic, nontherapeutic, or countertherapeutic" [Tomm 1987a, p. 4]. In this regard, the author relates an anecdote that was illuminating for him. During a couple therapy session, the partners talked about how much the situation had improved and how the level of conflict between them had decreased since they had started therapy. After a lively and amusing exchange about these changes, the therapist asked: "So what problems would you like to talk about today?". Following this seemingly innocuous question, the couple gradually moved towards an increasingly confrontational interaction. The author points out that he unfortunately did not consider then that instead of talking about problems he should have reinforced the new developments by asking questions aimed at supporting the recent changes [1987a]. Many questions have therapeutic effects on family members, both in a direct way through the implications of the questions, and in an indirect way through the verbal and non-verbal responses they receive from other family members. The role of the therapist is to conduct the session in such a way that the conversation becomes therapeutic. But the anecdote mentioned above shows that there are questions from the therapist that can even be non-therapeutic. Tomm's classification of questions [1985; 1987b; 1988] supports therapists in making decisions from time to time to create together with clients a new way of considering, evaluating, and explaining behaviours and events; and to support changes and resources expressed by them. Karl Tomm proposes four types of questions: linear, circular, strategic, and reflexive.

⇒ *Linear questions* are formulated to orient the therapist about the client's situation. Many interviews begin with at least a few linear questions. Often, this is necessary to approach clients through typical linear views of their problematic situation. For instance, the therapist may ask: *Why did you decide to come here today? Do you have any symptoms other than deep sadness?* This type of question tends to have a conservative effect, as people usually think of their problems in linear terms; therefore, linear questions introduce little "news of differences". Linear questions are necessary to develop an initial picture of the difficulty and are useful to establish an initial engagement. However, it is important to beware of their potential hazards, such as inadvertently funnelling the client towards even more linear perceptions, with implicit validation of pre-existing beliefs. For this reason, the recommendation is to integrate the exploration of the situation also with questions that solicit relational, systemic, and contextual descriptions, such as circular questions.

⇒ *Circular questions* "are formulated to bring forth the 'patterns that connect' persons, objects, actions, perceptions, ideas, feelings, events, beliefs, contexts, and so on, in recurrent or cybernetic circuits" [Tomm 1988, p. 7]. Circular questions can be formulated with the following intentions:

- Investigate how a third party (client) sees the relationship between 2 other family members;
- Identify the circumstances in which specific interactive behaviours are enacted;

- Highlight differences in interpersonal interaction within specific relationships;
- Formulate a ranking of positions of various family members with respect to a given behaviour or interaction;
- Detect changes in a relationship, before and after a specific event; and
- Stimulate reflection on the differences that might occur between the current situation and hypothetical scenarios.

Circular questions tend to be characterized by a general curiosity about the possible connections of the events surrounding the problem, rather than a need to know exactly where the problem originated.

Taking a circular perspective, a therapist might ask: *What does your father do when you and your mother quarrel? Who thinks you're not a good parent?*

Circular questions can have liberating effects on the client or family. While the therapist asks these questions to identify circular patterns and understand the situation from a systemic point of view, family members make their own connections by listening to the responses of those present or by imagining the responses of those who are evoked in the conversation. In this way, it is possible for them to become aware of the circularity of their interactive patterns. This increased awareness liberates clients from the limitations of their previous linear viewpoints and helps them address their own difficulties from a new perspective. A potential hazard in using circular questions is that as the therapist explores wider and wider areas of interaction, the conversation may drift towards areas that might seem irrelevant to clients' immediate needs and interests.

⇒ *Strategic questions* are an indirect way of giving suggestions or advice, e.g., *Have you ever thought of talking to your father about this? Since yelling hasn't worked for 20 years, have you ever thought of doing something else?* Strategic questions contain advice formulated in the terms of a question. Therefore, they do not bind clients to follow the given advice but leave them free to consider whether to follow it or not. Differently from direct advice, strategic questions do not imply judgement. These questions can be used to introduce different patterns of thinking and behaviour, without having to resort to direct statements or instructions. Because of their nature, too many strategic questions could have undesirable, counter-therapeutic effects. However, if accurately expressed, these questions can help clients to confront themselves with the limitations, constraints, and contradictions of their belief system and behaviours.

⇒ *Reflexive questions* assume that family members are autonomous individuals and cannot be instructed as robots. The most important premise underlying these questions is that the therapeutic system is co-evolutionary and that the therapist acts to encourage family members' reflection on their own belief systems and behaviours. Examples are as follows: *If your depression suddenly disappeared, how would your life change? If your partner will never change, how long are you willing to bear all that?* These questions are reflexive in that they are formulated to encourage clients to reflect on the implications of their usual perceptions and actions, and to consider new possibilities. There can be as many reflective questions as many hypotheses therapists can formulate about the distress or concerns of an individual, a couple, or a family, according to the strategies they considers useful to help the client find a different way to solve their problems. For example, reflexive questions can be divided as follows:

- Future-oriented questions: *If your husband continues to behave like this, how do you expect you will react?*
- Observer-perspective questions: *How did you interpret the situation that gave rise to these concerns?*
- Unexpected context-change questions: to a couple reporting continuous conflict, the therapist asks: *When was the last time the two of you had fun together?*
- Embedded-suggestion questions: *"If, instead of not saying anything and avoiding her, you admitted you made a mistake and apologized, what do you think might happen?"* [Tomm 1987b, p. 178].
- Normative comparison questions: *If you realized how common these problems are, would it be easier for you to talk about them?*
- Distinction-clarifying questions: *"What is really most important for you, being highly successful in your career or having a rich family life?"* [Tomm 1987b, p. 180].
- Questions introducing hypotheses: *In your opinion, is there a more useful way to help/distract your mother than to have difficulties at school?*
- Process-interruption questions: *"When your parents are at home, do they argue as much as they do here?"* [Tomm 1987b, p. 181].

Through reflective questions, clients are invited to consider new points of view; in doing so, they generate new connections and new solutions in their own way and at their own pace.

The questions described and classified by Tomm are to be considered as guidelines for the therapist's action. It is the therapist who evaluates on a moment-by-moment basis whether to ask a certain type of question, according to the feedback coming from the family members and the relational context that has been shaped.

Questions generating new perspectives

In addition to those described above, we present some types of questions that aim to create a generative context to stimulate clients toward the adoption of a different perspective to look at themselves and their significant others.

⇒ *Questions that encourage decentring* invite each interlocutor to focus on the Other's point of view, thus "seeing" that there may be different ways of understanding a behaviour or explaining an event. Usually, the therapist asks for the opinion of all family members about the various issues addressed, so everyone has the opportunity to hear the others' viewpoint. But this does not guarantee that everyone's points of view are considered. When that happens, the therapist may use questions that ask the interlocutor to assume the other's perspective, e.g., *What do you think your mother feels about ...? If I would ask Mary, what would she say?*

Systemic therapists adopt this style of conducting the interview also in individual therapies, when significant others are not physically present, but are evoked during the conversation [Boscolo and Bertrando 1996].

⇒ *Questions that encourage taking responsibility for one's own feelings, thinking, and actions.* By means of linguistic expedients, these questions allow the therapist to negotiate descriptions in which the individuals assume responsibility for their actions. As an example, let us consider an excerpt from an interview with Helen, who suffers because of a problematic relationship with her sister:

Therapist (to Helen):	Do you think that something should be done to solve this problem?
Helen:	I don't know. I've tried ... I'm bearing up, so I don't ... We cannot restore a relationship on that basis.
Therapist:	This means that you are willing to accept the relationship with your sister as it is ...
Helen:	Yes.
Therapist:	When did you become aware of this?
Helen:	Since I started feeling unwell.
Therapist:	When was that ...?
Helen:	Two years ago. Before that I struggled.
Therapist:	Did you try to change things before?
Helen:	Yes.
Therapist:	Then for the last 2 years...
Helen:	... that's it, it's over, there's nothing I can do...
Therapist:	.... . so, we can probably reflect on the consequences of staying in the relationship with your sister with the problems you see, without wanting to change her...
Helen:	... without *being able* to change her ... but I'm not feeling well.
Therapist:	Ah, so deep down you still want to change her.
Helen:	Probably.
Therapist:	Well, we'll work on this.

⇒ *Questions that recognize the interlocutor's competence.* The therapist interacts with the clients assuming that everyone can answer the questions and that all answers are legitimate [Peräkylä *et al.* 2008]. Therefore, she creates space for everyone to express their views, explores everyone's ideas, and prevents some opinions from being disqualified. Let us consider an example from the excerpt of a family therapy interview:

Therapist: How did the other therapies end?
Albert: I realize now that I did not enjoy my youth very much. I am touchy and to be taken with a grain of salt. But if one succeeds in creating a relationship, I am a faithful lapdog.
Father: I know why he interrupted therapies.
Therapist: Albert knows it too!
Albert: I really don't know why, but maybe because I lived them badly. Now I can say that it was a wrong attitude ... . I do not consider these experiences as failures.

⇒ *Questions that call for coherence between apparently contradictory facts.* Identify contradictions in what the clients say is a privileged way of constructing descriptions, explanations, or meanings of the family's situation, and finding possible solutions together with the family members. To do so, therapists may ask questions that Viaro and Leonardi [1983] define as "corrective". With these questions, the therapist collects some information that the family members have provided, juxtaposes them, and points out that they do not match. In the interpersonal process of coherence reconstruction, family members develop a new position.

Here is an example from a family therapy interview:

Therapist: (talking to the father) Where do you think Mia got the idea of having to take care of your and your wife's problems?
Father: Because she has a great deal of imagination.
Therapist: Is there anyone who asks her to do so?
Father: It may also be the religious thing. It is a fact that she had a physical and mental breakdown after a pilgrimage to Lourdes. She came home skinny, changed ... .
Therapist: That is, far from home.
Father: Not just any far from home, a particular far from home. When she came home from Lourdes, it was like having a saint in the house. She was clearing the table, using a tone of voice that ... she was washing dishes. She became so good, even too good. She almost scared me.
Therapist: What stands out to me is that even Henry, who has no religious ideas, felt at some point in his life that he had to do something for the 2 of you.

This type of intervention can also be structured in the form of a paraphrase, recalling the interventions made by family members, e.g., *Miriam, I still don't understand what your husband's strictness consists of. On one hand your children say that if they want to go out, they must ask Dad because he always says yes, while Mom says to stay at home. But then they all say that Dad is stricter. So, what does your husband's strictness consist of?*

⇒ *Response-based questions.* In therapy with people who have experienced violence or abuse, questions about the effects of violence put the subject in a passive position, as a powerless victim. On the contrary, questions about how they responded and resisted violence or abuse put the subject in an active position, of competence and agency [Coates and Wade 2004; Davolo and Mancini 2017]. Instead of focusing the story on the abuser and the effects of the abuse, the focus is on how the abused tried to resist or react, e.g., *What did you do when your boss threatened you for the first time? Where were you when the robbers snatched your mother's handbag, and what did you do? How did you react when your uncle tried to trap you and forced you to touch him?*

⇒ *Questions about a hypothetical audience.* Gail Simon [1998] coined this term to describe a group of people who are not physically present, but whose stories have similarities with the client's situation. Questions about the hypothetical audience help to build a context of belonging to which the client can imagine turning to for support, advice, stories, and resources. For example: *If you were to ask other parents who have raised a severely disabled child, with a story just like yours, what advice would they give you in this situation? If you were to tell your story to other people who have recently moved to this country as refugees, what might they perceive about your state of mind at this moment in your relationship, where one of you is completely satisfied with her job and the other completely frustrated?* The use of hypothetical audiences has proved useful when clients rigidly describe their difficulties in a decontextualized way, and/or when clients present themselves as isolated, with no peer group and no community to draw on for advice or support.

The main characteristic of the systemic technical interventions is that they do not provide different points of view or different solutions; rather, they prompt family members to generate for themselves a different point of view. The preeminent aim is not for the subjects to abandon a way of thinking in favour of one that the therapist considers more appropriate, but to break the rigidity of the clients' patterns of reference and trigger a process of change.

Therapeutic practices for narrative changes

According to Sluzki [1992], the ultimate goal of a therapeutic encounter is to produce transformations in clients' dominant stories, because the way the problem is described and explained is also the way the problem is experienced.

Clients' stories may have rigid contents and structures that leave no space for change; the role of therapy is to enable clients' stories to become more flexible. That is why during the interviews the therapist explores how the story is organized and how it develops, and through questions and comments the therapist tries to introduce transformations both in the content and in the way the story is narrated. Through the dialogue between the therapist and clients, new characters, plot, and developments are introduced. As it combines in a different way components of the old story, the story that emerges from the therapeutic conversations is a new one. Therapists must introduce perturbations within the narrative structure proposed by the participants to favour a shift in the way clients talk about problems, consequences, and possible solutions. Fostering new stories can be done through "transformative micro-practices", which consist of questions and comments directed at redefining or clarifying what is proposed in the narrative [*ibidem*]. Transformative micro-practices may concern the narrative dimensions that characterize the content of the story (*transformations in the nature of the story*), or the dimensions that characterize the structure of the narrative, i.e., the way in which clients position themselves in the narrative (*transformations in the telling of the story*) (see Table 2.1).

The dimensions defining the content of a story are: time (events or behaviours are narrated as stable vs changing); space (events and behaviours are contextualized or not); causality (the emphasis is on the origins vs effects of actions and events); interactions (the story is centred on intra-personal vs inter-personal aspects); and values (events and behaviours are described as legitimate vs illegitimate). The dimensions of the narrative's structure concern the extent to which the clients describe themselves as *passive* or *active* in relation to events, prefer *descriptions* or *interpretations*, and present themselves and others as *competent* or *incompetent*.

Table 2.1 Transformative therapeutic micro-practices [Sluzki 1992, p. 222]

TRANSFORMATIONS	
Dimensions	Shifts
In Time	Static/Fluctuating
	Nouns/Verbs
	Ahistoric/Historic
In Space	Noncontextual/Contextual
In Causality	Cause/Effects
In Interactions	Intra-/Interpersonal
	Intentions/Effects
	Symptoms/Conflicts
	Roles/Rules
In Values	Good Intent/Bad Intent
	Sane/Insane
	Legitimate/Illegitimate
In the Telling	Passive/Active
	Interpretations/Descriptions
	Incompetence/Competence

Clients' stories are rigid if these dimensions are exclusively positioned on either one or the other pole. Transformative micro-practices then are meant to shift the story to the opposite pole through questions or comments. Let us see them in detail.

Transformations in the nature of stories

Transformations in the nature of the story may concern time, space, causality, interactions, and values.

⇒   Transformations in *time* can be:

Static/Fluctuating: when clients describe the problem as a stable or unchangeable phenomenon, the therapist introduces fluctuating transformations. Time fluctuations can enhance the description of exceptions and alternative scenarios. For example: *In which moments did you happen not to argue?* The opposite transformation is useful when the narrative is a succession of events and circumstances without a constant condition. Together with the client the therapist identifies a connection between the many descriptions produced, as in the following example: *If we were to find a common thread for all these aspects you have described, what would it be?*

Nouns/Verbs: the therapist proposes transformations from nouns to verbs to introduce the difference between the characteristics of people and the characteristics of actions when clients describe people or situations having unchanging characteristics, e.g., *What are the behaviours of your partner that lead you to define her/him as hostile?* The opposite transformation, from verbs to nouns, is useful when the client proposes a sequence of actions without drawing a general categorization. For example: *How would you define your mother in relation to the behaviours you have described?*

Ahistoric/Historic: these transformations refer to the transition from a story in which there are no temporal references to one with a specific starting point, a given scenario and an evolution. In those cases, the therapist may ask, e.g., *When did this begin?* The introduction of a temporal and contextual dimension allows the client to identify exceptions and alternative models to the narrated story. The opposite transformation is useful when the aim is to highlight alternatives to a symptomatic stalemate characterized by a story in which all the responsibility is assigned to past circumstances. For example: *You are saying that your problems have been present for several years. Why did you decide to seek professional help now?*

⇒ Transformations in *space* involve a shift from a *noncontextual* to a *contextual* narrative, and vice versa. Introducing the spatial dimension makes it possible to consider the framework of a circumstance and the mutual influence that context and event have in the telling of a story. For example: *Under which circumstances do you most frequently experience the discomfort you are talking about?*

Conversely, shifting the focus from the context to the event serves to highlight its characteristics: *Now that you have moved to a new house, how can you explain the fact that the 2 of you are still arguing?*

⇒ Transformations in *causality* involve a shift from *cause* to *effects*, and vice versa. When the client's story is focused exclusively on events described as the causes and origins of the problem, it is useful for the therapist to shift the narrative to the effects of those events, e.g., *In which way do you think that the divorce of your parents could influence your current problems in your relationship?* Conversely, when the client dwells too much on the effects of a problem, the therapist may ask questions about the origins of the problem, to explore clients' point of view about causes. For example: *When did this long period of difficulty begin? What was happening at that time in your family?* These questions may let ideas emerge about justifications and responsibilities that could be then destabilized by exploring the opposite direction.

⇒   Transformations in *interactions* are grouped into 4 subcategories:

Intra-Personal/Inter-Personal: these transformations refer to the shift from a story centred on a person or a situation in terms of attributes, to one in which the descriptions concern patterns of interactions between 2 or more people. When the clients' story is centred on the properties of an individual, the therapist can redirect the narrative through interpersonal transformation, as in the following example: *Considering your dedication, how do you see the relationship between you and your partner: equal or unbalanced?* On the other hand, if a story emphasises mainly the interactive patterns, it is useful to introduce an intrapersonal transformation, which can provide a new type of description focused on personal qualities. The therapist may ask, for instance, *Do these behaviours make you think of your daughter as a loner?*

Intentions/Effects: turning a story centred on a person's intentions into one centred on the effects of a behaviour can help weaken the attribution of negative intent of others, e.g., *You say that your father is not interested in you, but how did you feel when you received his phone call?* On the other hand, the opposite transformation is proposed when the therapist's intention is to try to understand the intentions that provoked a certain effect. For example: *What led you to scold your son so harshly?*

Symptoms/Conflicts: When the client's narrative is too symptom-centred, the therapist can help by shifting the focus of the story to the reciprocal effects between the patient's behaviour and that of others. A symptom-focused narrative is a story centred on the difficulties of 1 individual, therefore moving the conversation on the conflict side allows for showing the reciprocal effects of all behaviours, opening the way to different perspectives and to a reflection on the cause–effect dynamics of the event. The therapist might inquire: *When you feel bad, how do your family members react?* A transformation in the opposite direction is proposed by the therapist when the clients focus too much on the reciprocal behaviours, neglecting the symptom manifested by themself or by others. The therapist may ask, for instance, *How can you expect to have a good time with your partner if she is depressed?*

Roles/Rules: a role-centred narrative deprives the story of the interpersonal dynamic of which that role is a part. The transformation from roles to rules "adds context, re-shuffles responsibilities, enriches the scenario" [Sluzki 1992, p. 225]. For example, when dealing with a narrative that puts the son in the role of arrogant, the therapist might ask: *Does your husband also consider your son's behaviour as arrogant?* The opposite transformation makes it possible to use the roles recognized by our culture to highlight different positions and bring out unexplored variables, e.g., *By behaving in this way, you play the role of the father, and who assumes the role of the son?*

⇒ Transformations in the *value* of the story are grouped into 3 subcategories:

Good intent/Bad intent: the transformation that emphasises good intentions allows the problematic behaviour to be redefined with a positive connotation. For example, if a daughter is described by her parents as confrontational, the therapist may ask, *From whom did your daughter learn to be so determined in her positions?*

Sane/Insane: this transformation makes it possible to move from rigid attributions of craziness to an attribution of saneness so that the story can be seen from another perspective, setting aside the alibi of madness. For example, if a client reports that they go crazy when taking drugs, the therapist may comment, *What you said when you were drugged may not have sounded kind, but it makes sense to me.*

Legitimate/Illegitimate: the terms legitimate/illegitimate are used as synonyms for reasonable/unreasonable and logical/illogical. This transformation makes it possible to redefine the value of an event, and to label the behaviour in negative or positive terms, to generate new interpretations and new implications. This is the case in [Sluzki's 1992, p. 226] example: "a woman, in the course of her consultation describes, with indignation, that her mother told her that they wouldn't get along if they were to live together at this time. The therapist's comment, *A rather lucid lady, your mother!* (in a context of trust) shatters the implicit assumption of agreement about the mother's unreasonableness".

Transformations in the telling of the story

Transformations in the *telling of the story* are of 3 types:

⇒ *Passive/Active*: the shift from a passive to an active narration allows the subject to take responsibility for their actions and to expand the stories. When clients describe a situation in which they present themself as a victim of another person or an event, the therapist may ask, *For how long do you think you will be able to accept this situation?* However, as Sluzki [1992] points out, the passive stance may be difficult to be modified in stories where the actor is a person in a fragile condition who suffers for a lack of alternatives (e.g., a frail elderly person, a person suffering a chronic pain). In these cases, supporting at first the passive position can be useful to empower the subject and encourage the acquisition of an active role later in the development of the therapeutic process.

⇒ *Interpretations/Descriptions*: when the subject has underlying beliefs about hidden meanings of certain events, it is useful for the therapist to ask for a more detailed description of those events. For example: *But what happened when − as you said − your relationship had "crystallised"?* If the descriptions overlook the underlying intentions of a particular behaviour, the therapist can encourage the client to provide an interpretation by asking questions such as: *And what do you think about all these events that happened to you?*

⇒ *Incompetence/Competence*: if clients describe themself as incompetent, the therapist can shift the narrative to the axis of competence, for example, by emphasising positive characteristics or attributes of the subject, e.g., *I think you have been very sensitive in realizing what was happening.* The opposite transformation is useful when the therapist deliberately wants to bring out a certain degree of weakness in individuals who present a flawless image of themselves. The therapist may comment, *Even strong people like you hide weaknesses; otherwise they could not be considered as strong.*

Sluzki's transformative micro-practices provide a map for moving into the territory of therapies, and for enriching and broadening the therapist's conversational skills. However, as for any other conceptual tool, the author stresses the importance of using this model on an instrumental, and not on a subservient basis. He reminds us that: "what many expert therapists call 'intuition' may consist precisely in having learned and then forgotten the right things!" [1992, p. 229].

Observational, metaphoric, and narrative tools

Conversational tools do not cover all the technical background of the systemic/constructionist/dialogical therapist. Other tools can be used during a session when the conversation guided by questions does not provide a helpful understanding of the situation; or when it is necessary to rely on more analogical or interactive tools such as narrative, observational, and metaphorical ones to favour a transformative dialogue, to encourage self-reflexivity and the construction of a shared context, thus letting new meanings and new stories emerge.

Among the *narrative techniques* the Family Life Chronology [Satir 1964] and the Genogram [McGoldrick, Gerson and Petry 2020; de Bernart and Merlini 2001] are to be mentioned. The *Family life chronology* consists of a semi-structured interview that, through circular questions, allows to recall the most important events in the life of the family (deaths, marriages, births, transfers, etc.) and to collect information about the marital relationship, the rules, and the family patterns. According to Satir, when used in the first few sessions, this technique can alleviate the initial fear and anxiety, help gathering information to attribute a meaning to the symptom, and instil hope in the clients.

The *Genogram* is a method to investigate and analyze family history to understand and give meaning to events. According to a precise symbolism, clients draw themself and the members of their family, including information about at least 3 generations. This provides a drawing of family life through which the story of the family is narrated. Acting as a guide, the therapist proposes questions and comments to help the clients identify and understand various patterns in their family history that may have an influence on a current issue. Although the genogram as a drawing of the family tree is a standardized method used by many therapists, there are multiple ways to work with this representation in the therapeutic conversation which, with a few exceptions [de Bernart and Merlini 2001; Schutzenberger 2014], are often left to the creativity of the clinician.

Among the *observational techniques*, T.I.A.P. (*Triadic Interaction Analytical Procedure*) [Venturelli *et al.* 2016] is an observational procedure for triadic interactions. Through the analysis of family interactions during a semi-structured game, this procedure identifies some family relational patterns that can support the hypothesizing process; in particular, how do family members deal with changes, how do they re-construct stability, how do they cope with separations during family microtransitions, and how are they coordinated in carrying on these processes. The results of this observational analysis are connected to what has emerged so far in the therapeutic dialogue about the family story. T.I.A.P. is employed in the psychotherapeutic field, but recently it has proved to be useful also in the field of parenting assessment. In that context, the procedure detects elements of family functioning, highlighting problems but also resources that are useful to identify, if necessary, the most appropriate intervention for the recovery of parenting [Venturelli, Fruggeri and Cigala 2022].

Metaphorical techniques include *Family Sculpting* [Duhl, Kantor and Duhl 1973]. This technique consists of portraying a spatial representation of the family or the couple. One or more members of the family arrange the others in relation to one another in the space. After the "sculpture of the family" has been realized, it is "fixed" by leaving it in the space for a significant amount of time. Then, family members discuss the feelings it has evoked in them. When making a sculpture, movement can also be introduced to emphasize certain sequences of interaction. It is also possible to introduce the temporal dimension [Onnis *et al.* 1994] by asking each family member to portray the family system in 3 specific phases of their life cycle: the present, the past, and the future.

The analogical and interactive techniques described above can be adapted to different cultural forms, social arrangements, and "families of choice" (non-hetero-normative).

The tools described in this chapter have different functions in the construction of the therapeutic dialogue; in this sense, their use cannot leave out the therapist's analysis of the dialogical and relational context that has been structured with a specific client. The therapists evaluate which instrument to choose according to the assessment they make of the dialogical context. With clients presenting a rigid narrative, the therapist will adopt the transformative practices suggested by Sluzki. If clients propose linear descriptions of their situation, therapists will rely on circular questions. When the therapists observe a lack of decentring to the other's point of view, they will support clients in developing mutual attention, with the discursive practices suggested by different authors or with the questions proposed by Brown. When the client appears to be particularly lacking in social or community resources, the evocation of the hypothetical audience conceived by Gail Simon can be a resource for change. However, if the verbal channel proves to be inadequate to introduce differences, the therapist will turn to analogue tools. The description of the various questions and the indication of their function in the conversational context constitute a knowledge available to therapists, who will use it being aware that questions are dialogical tools whose usefulness is ultimately confirmed only by the clients' feedback.

References

Boscolo, L. and Bertrando, P. [1996], *Systemic therapy with individuals*, London, Routledge.

Brown, E. [1997], *The question cube: a model for developing question repertoire in training couple and family therapists*, in Journal of Family Marital Therapy, 23, 1, pp. 27–40.

Byrne, N. and McCarthy, I. [2007], *The dialectical structure of hope and despair: a fifth province approach*, in C. Flaskas, I. McCarthy and J. Sheehan (eds.), *Hope and despair in narrative and family therapy: reflections on adversity, forgiveness and reconciliation*, Hove/NY, Brunner Routledge, pp. 36–48.

Coates, L. and Wade, A. [2004] *Telling it like it isn't: obscuring perpetrator responsibility for violent crime*, in Discourse and Society, 15, 5, pp. 499–526.

Davolo, A. and Mancini, T. [2017], *L'intervento psicologico con i migranti*, Bologna, Il Mulino.

de Bernart, R. and Merlini, F. [2001], *Una bibliografia ragionata su: il genogramma familiare*, in Terapia Familiare, 65, pp.77–101.

Duhl, F.J., Kantor, D. and Duhl, B. [1973], *Learning space, and action in family therapy: a primer of sculpture*, in Seminars in Psychiatry, 5, pp. 167–183.

Fleuridas, C., Nelson, T. and Rosenthal, D. [1986], *The evolution of circular questions: training family therapists*, in Journal of Marital and Family Therapy, 12, 2, pp. 113–127.

McCarthy, I. and Byrne, N. [1988], *Mistaken love: conversations on the problem of incest in an Irish context*, in Family Process, 27, pp. 181–199.

McGoldrick, M., Gerson, R. and Petry, S.S. [2020], *Genograms: assessment and intervention*, New York, WW Norton & Company.

Onnis, L., Gennaro, A.D., Cespa, G., Agostini, B., Chouhy, A., Dentale, R.C. and Quinzi, P. [1994], *Sculpting present and future: a systemic intervention model applied to psychosomatic families*, in Family Process, 33, 3, pp. 341–355.

Penn, P. [1982], *Circular questioning*, in Family Process, 21, pp. 267–280.

Penn, P. [1985], *Feed-forward: future questions, future maps*, in Family Process, 24, pp. 299–311.

Peräkylä, A.E., Antaki, C.E., Vehviläinen, S.E. and Leudar, I.E. [2008], *Conversation analysis and psychotherapy*, Cambridge, Cambridge University Press.

Satir, V. [1964], *Conjoint family therapy*, Palo Alto CA, Science and Behavior Books.

Schutzenberger, A.A. [2014], *The ancestor syndrome: transgenerational psychotherapy and the hidden links in the family tree*, London, Routledge.

Simon, G. [1998], *Incitement to riot? Individual identity and group membership: some reflections on the politics of a post-modernist therapy*, in Human Systems, 9, 1, pp. 33–50.

Sluzki, C. [1992], *Transformations: a blueprint for narrative changes in therapy*, in Family Process, 31, pp. 217–230.

Tomm, K. [1985], *Circular interviewing: a multifaceted clinical tool*, in D. Campbell and R. Draper (eds), *Applications of systemic family therapy*, London, Grune and Stratton, pp. 33–45.

Tomm, K. [1987a], *Interventive interviewing: part I. Strategizing as a fourth guideline for the therapist*, in Family Process, 26, pp. 3–13.

Tomm, K. [1987b], *Interventive interviewing: part II. Reflexive questioning as a means to enable self-healing*, in Family Process, 26, pp. 167–183.

Tomm, K. [1988], *Interventive interviewing: part III. Intending to ask linear, circular, strategic or reflexive questions*, in Family Process, 27, pp. 1–15.

Venturelli, E., Cabrini, E., Fruggeri, L. and Cigala, A. [2016], *The study of triadic family interactions: the proposal of an observational procedure*, in Integrative Psychological Behavioral Science, 50, 4, pp. 655–683.

Venturelli, E., Fruggeri, L. and Cigala, A. [2022], *Valutazione del funzionamento familiare. La prospettiva triadica della procedura TIAP*, Milano: Raffaello Cortina.

Viaro, M. and Leonardi, P. [1983], *Getting and giving information: analysis of a family-interview strategy*, in Family Process, 22, 1, pp. 27–42.

Part II

Relational competency: promoting and analyzing intersubjectivity

3 The therapeutic alliance

The scientific literature has extensively documented that the quality of the client–therapist relationship is central to the success of psychotherapeutic interventions: it is through relationships that interventions are deployed and become effective. Summarizing evidences on the effectiveness of psychotherapies, Fife and colleagues [2014] elaborated the Therapeutic Pyramid (see Introduction), which iconically illustrates how technical competency is implemented through the relationship that develops between therapist and client. Consistently, the technical competency described in the previous chapter cannot be detached from the relational competency, namely therapists' ability to analyze and monitor the interactive relational process that unfolds between them and clients.

The definition of *therapeutic relationship* is twofold: on the one hand, it refers to the quality of the relationship created between therapist and client; on the other hand, it refers to the meaning-making process that the therapist and clients co-create through their interaction. More specifically, the first definition concerns the quality and strength of the collaborative relationship developed between the client and therapist, and the ability to negotiate the objectives and tasks of the treatment: in the contexts of research and intervention, all this is known as the therapeutic alliance. From this point of view, the relational competency of psychotherapists refers to the ability to create a good alliance and to monitor the development of the alliance during the psychotherapeutic process. The second definition of the therapeutic relationship concerns the construction of meanings that therapists and clients negotiate through their interactions. In this sense, the relational competency refers to the therapists' ability to observe how the therapist and clients engage in the co-construction of meanings, identities, relationships, and social realities in order to position themself to facilitate the creation of transformative contexts. In this chapter, we discuss the therapeutic relationship in terms of therapeutic alliance, whereas in the next chapter we will focus on the meaning-making interactive process.

DOI: 10.4324/9781003278092-6

Therapeutic alliance in individual, couple, and family therapies

Change, interruption, or continuation of therapy depend, to some extent, on clients' perception of how much the therapist cares for them [Friedlander, Escudero and Heatherington 2006]. The collaborative relationship between the therapist and client created during psychotherapy sessions is defined as "alliance". This term stresses that therapeutic relationships should be characterized by mutual trust, sympathy, respect, and care, as well as agreement on the goals of the therapy and a commitment to work together for their achievement [Horvath and Bedi 2002]. A good relationship between the therapist and client is the core element of a successful therapy. Several research studies have shown that amongst the different aspects that define therapeutic relationships, alliance is the main predictor of positive outcomes for individual therapy [Horvath and Symonds 1991; Martin, Garske and Davis 2000], couples therapy [Johnson and Talitman 1997; Quinn, Dotson and Jordan 1997; Knobloch-Fedders, Pinsof and Mann 2007], and family therapy [Johnson, Wright and Ketring 2002; Escudero *et al.* 2008]. Furthermore, when therapeutic alliance is undermined, clients tend to interrupt therapies prematurely [Sharf, Primavera and Diener 2010; Yoo, Bartle-Haring and Gangamma 2016].

For many years, the construct of therapeutic alliance has been associated with the different orientations of psychodynamic approaches; in the 1970s, its centrality for any psychotherapeutic treatment, regardless the orientation, has been acknowledged [Strupp 1973]. Bordin [1979] was the first to integrate different theoretical contributions concerned with therapeutic alliance and to develop a definition that is still relevant for both individual and couple/family therapy. According to this author [ibidem], the definition of therapeutic alliance entails: an agreement between the therapist and client on the objectives of the treatment, an agreement on the tasks necessary for the achievement of the therapeutic aims, and an emotional bond between the 2. This definition emphasizes 2 central aspects of the therapist–client relationship: the involvement of the latter in the therapeutic process in terms of collaboration, and the emotional connection needed to favour the therapeutic change. Bordin's [ibidem] definition has received wide recognition from the scientific community to the extent that most methods used to assess therapeutic alliance both in individual and conjoint therapy are based on this conceptualization.

Although the agreement on the goals and tasks of the therapy and the emotional bond between the client and therapist are central aspects in every therapeutic context, it is important to differentiate between individual therapy and conjoint (couple or family) therapy. In individual therapy, clients contact a practitioner, negotiate what to share of themself and the persons they relate to, decide what to keep and what to reject of what the professional says, and develop a particular emotional relationship. By contrast, in conjoint therapy the co-presence of several people with different points of view limits individual freedom and control over the situation, thereby making the construction of a positive alliance much more complex. Firstly, in conjoint therapy, what family members say and the relationship they create with the therapist occurs in the presence of others [Pinsof and Catherall 1986]. Therefore, the therapeutic alliance includes not only the client and the therapist, but also the therapist and the other family members as well as the relationships among all family members [Pinsof 1994; 1995]. These different alliances are not separated; rather, they influence each other. Friedlander and colleagues [2006, p. 20] have pointed out that to work effectively with couples and families, "the therapist must figure out how to nurture alliances with multiple clients whose working capacities, personalities, developmental needs, and clinical issues are likely to differ", while looking at the needs of the single individuals and of the group as a whole. However, even this is not enough: another crucial aspect to consider in couple and family therapy is clients' safety; namely, clients should feel comfortable enough to talk about their relationships, without fearing of being blamed or denigrated for what they say both during the therapeutic session and afterwards in the post-session. In a nutshell, clients should feel that there will be no consequences for what they say during the therapy encounters [Friedlander *et al.* 2006].

Therapeutic alliance is continuously fostered by the contribution of all participants in the therapy session. Therapeutic alliance needs to be monitored constantly because despite an initial positive bond, clients' disappointment at the therapist's apparent lack of understanding of their problems can emerge at any moment and lead to the interruption of the therapy [Beck, Friedlander and Escudero 2006]. Drop-out and split alliances are not uncommon (see Box 3.1). A good alliance is not built once and for all, but it is the outcome of a dynamic process characterized by interruptions and repairs.

Box 3.1   Split alliance and drop out

The term "breaking the alliance" indicates a moment in which, during the therapeutic process, the collaboration between the client and therapist is particularly difficult. In general terms, both in individual and in conjoint therapies, the breakdown of the therapeutic alliance is manifested through withdrawal, or the absence of involvement in the therapy, or through an explicit disagreement with the therapist. When there is more than 1 client, as in the case of couple or family therapies, the breaking of the alliance can also take the form of a split. A split alliance occurs when there are significant differences between family members in the attitude towards therapy, in terms of goals and tasks, or towards the therapist [Friedlander *et al.* 2006]. This divergence takes on an even more problematic connotation when the feelings of some are accompanied by the antagonism of others [Pinsof 1995]. There are many reasons that can lead to a split. In fact, it can derive from the therapist's loss of impartiality, from a therapist's failure to recognize a hierarchy within the family, from the fear of some clients of being blamed, from a triangulation of the therapist in family dynamics, and more [Pinsof 1994; Beck *et al.* 2006; Escudero and Friedlander 2017].

Considering the family as a system, empathizing with everyone, and identifying therapeutic goals that involve all members are the ways to prevent the dynamics that can lead to split alliance. However, in the event of a split occurring, it is important to be able to recognize and repair it. The reparation can be done by talking about what is happening, if the break is explicit; through the search for an emotional connection or through indirect interventions that involve other family members in support of those who at the moment appear to be in difficulty with the therapeutic context [Friedlander *et al.* 1994]. An alliance can be considered repaired if the client exhibits behaviours that indicate a positive alliance with the therapist and the other family members, if the therapist and client deal with the breakdown of the alliance directly or indirectly, and finally if both succeed in moving on and resume a collaboration with respect to the objectives of the treatment [Escudero *et al.* 2012]. The breaking of an alliance cannot always be repaired. When this is not possible, the most frequent outcome is drop-out: the patient's choice to prematurely interrupt the undertaken psychotherapeutic process [Yoo *et al.* 2016].

The SOFTA model for the study of therapeutic alliance

The System for Observing Family Therapy Alliances (SOFTA) is a conceptual model elaborated by Friedlander, Escudero and Heatheringotn [2006] and originated from the creation of observational (SOFTA-o) and self-report (SOFTA-s) tools[1] for evaluating the strength of the therapeutic alliance in the context of couple and family therapy.

The empirical validation of methods to assess therapeutic alliance indicates that it can be reliably measured through both self-report questionnaires administered to clients and therapists, and observational tools used by external observers. Self-reports allow for the collection of clients' points of view; this is crucial to the treatment, since clients' perception of the therapeutic alliance is the strongest predictor of the therapeutic success [Horvath and Symonds 1991]. However, relying on self-report evaluations only has limitations since they cannot provide information about the clients' and therapists' behaviours that enable the development of a trustful relationship. On the contrary, having such information, therapists could adopt methods and techniques that could improve a compromised alliance. SOFTA allows therapists to overcome this limitation, proposing the assessment of alliances also through observational tools: both clients' and therapist's contribution to the creation of the therapeutic alliance can be identified through indicators of positive or negative verbal and non-verbal behaviours. SOTFA's authors have developed the observational indicators through a systematic literature review, clinical experience, and analysis of video-recorded therapy sessions.

The conceptualization of alliance proposed by the SOFTA model is trans-theoretical, interpersonal, and multidimensional. In other words, it is not grounded in a specific couple or family therapy approach; therefore, it pre-serves the "common factor" aspect of psychotherapy. Furthermore, SOFTA is interpersonal since it takes into account the actual interactions between the members of the family and between each member and the therapist. Lastly, it is a multidimensional model, since the construct of alliance is defined through 4 dimensions: *Engagement in the Therapeutic Process:* clients viewing the treatment as meaningful, a sense of being involved in therapy and working together with the therapist. *Emotional Connection to the Therapist:* clients viewing the therapist as an important person in their life, and a sense that the relationship is based on affiliation, trust, caring, and concern. *Safety within the Therapeutic System:* the client viewing therapy as a place to take risks, be open, be vulnerable, be flexible, feel a sense of comfort, and have an expectation that new experiences and learning will take place. *Shared Sense of Purpose within the Family:* family members seeing themselves as working collaboratively in therapy to improve family re-lations and achieve common family goals; moreover, a sense of solidarity in relation to the therapy ("we're in this together") [Friedlander *et al.* 2006, p. 216]. The 4 dimensions of the SOFTA are interdependent (see Figure 3.1): each of them highlights specific aspects of the therapeutic alliance, which cannot be separated from the others. The Engagement in the Therapeutic Process and the Emotional Connection to the Therapist refer to the client–therapist relationship and overlap with the characteristics of the therapeutic alliance identified by Bordin [1979]. The Safety within the Therapeutic System and the Shared Sense of Purpose within the Family concern family relationships and the family–therapist relationship, and are dimensions characterizing the therapeutic alliance in conjoint therapies. Additionally, Engagement and

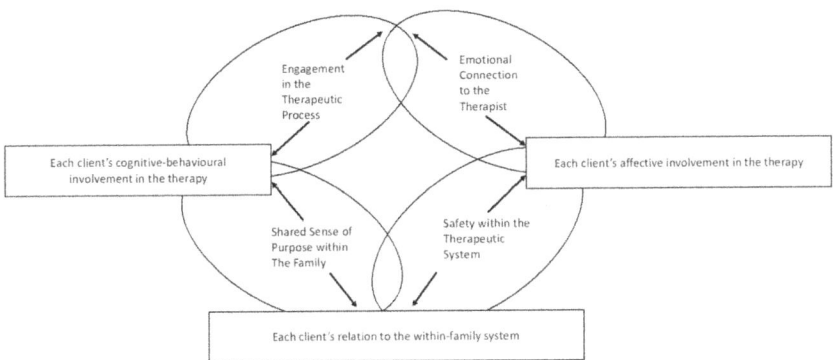

Figure 3.1 Interrelations of SOFTA dimensions [Friedlander, Escudero and Heatherington 2006, p. 40].

Shared Sense of Purpose address the cognitive-behavioural functioning, whereas Emotional Connection and Safety refers to emotional functioning. Given the interdependence among the 4 dimensions, the behaviours related to each SOFTA dimension reverberates on the other dimensions, thereby influencing the family alliance, and the alliance between each family member and the therapist. As an example for dimensions' interdependence, we can consider a therapy session in which a family member tells something unknown to the other members. According to the items of the SOFTA, this behaviour signals the client's sense of safety within the therapeutic system (including both the client–therapist relationship and the family members' relationships); this can trigger family members' perception of the therapy having a positive effect, which in turn activates the engagement of all family members in the therapy, thereby fostering the emotional connection (see Figure 3.1).

According to Escudero and Friedlander [2017], a clinical practice based on strong and solid family member alliances and client–therapist alliance should consider the role of the 4 dimensions across the therapy sessions. The first step to ensure the creation of good alliances is to provide clients with a minimum level of Safety, which can happen by stressing the relevance of privacy and acknowledging the understandable clients' difficulties in sharing private issues with a therapist. This favours the creation of a non-defensive context in which the Emotional Connection to the Therapist can be fostered. Acknowledging the subjective experience of every family member, as well as showing a genuine interest in the different points of view even when contrasting, prevent clients from feeling judged and foster the creation of emotional connection. Good Emotional Connection together with Safety, namely clients viewing the therapist as able to understand their emotional experiences and to protect them from further sufferings, allows clients to actively engage in the therapy. This means that clients feel they can take the risk to both openly talk about their problems and distress, and engage in the transformative process entailed in psychotherapy. Clients' engagement in the therapeutic process can be sustained by therapists' ability to convey the idea that therapy will help them change through the focus on small objectives and tasks, which will be achieved gradually. Nonetheless, in order to favour change in a family system, thereby making a therapy effective, family members should not only feel safe, emotionally connected, and actively engaged in the therapy process, but they should also feel united in reaching a common therapeutic goal. The creation of a shared sense of purpose within the family is a systemic therapeutic objective that can be achieved by underlining what family members have in common, such as feeling, points of view, and behaviours.

Safety within the therapeutic system

The SOFTA dimension of Safety refers to how much clients feel the therapy as a safe context in which they can take risks, be open, vulnerable, and flexible;

a context in which clients feel no need to be defensive because they perceive that conflict and dissent within the family can be expressed and handled without harm.

Different clues should make therapists aware that therapy might not be a safe place for clients: manifestation of anxiety, posture, avoiding visual contact with family members, and defensive answers can signal that clients fear therapy [Friedlander *et al.* 2006]. In individual therapies, clients can decide to show their vulnerabilities and disclose sensitive matters regarding their lives and identities. By contrast, in family therapies, members can fear the negative reactions of the others if they disclose something, or other family members could reveal something about other members, making them look bad. Family hostility, namely high level of conflict among family members, makes disclosure and engagement in the process of change more difficult. Therefore, fostering Safety entails identifying clients' signs of vulnerability; controlling the emergence of hostility, guilt, and contempt within the family; and containing symmetrical escalations and crossed blaming [Gottman 1994]. In some situations, the lack of Safety can be amplified by the intervention of social institutions, such as juvenile court and social services, that oblige families to start psychotherapy, as in the case example that follows.

The Murphy family contacts a private family therapy centre at the recommendation of the social worker, who has assisted the family for the problematic behaviour of their 15-year-old son, Nick. He has been sent to residential child care service after being involved in robberies that affected his peers and for drug dealing. Social workers have reported the situation to the Juvenile Court, describing Nick's family as a negative context for him, defining the parents as unable to help Nick take responsibility for his actions. The therapist invites the whole family to the first interview: the parents, Sarah and Sean; the eldest son, Sam, who is 19; and Nick. The parents appear quite frightened about what is happening in their family and painfully recall the moment when the police rang the bell to take Nick, without giving them the opportunity to prepare for that event. They describe their family as normal; both parents work as employees and claim they have always been present in their children's lives. The older son, Sam, has never caused troubles. He has studied and practiced sports, with very good results. Sean, the father, wants to make a good impression on the therapist: he acts as the spokesperson of the family, detailing all the legal actions they have taken to assist with Nick's issues. The mother, Sarah, looks submissive but supportive of her husband: she is suffering for her son's behaviour; she says: "He is not the kid he used to be". When invited to express his point of view, Sam says he would have never expected Nick to do what he did, given the way they have been raised. While Nick is listening to his family members' point of view, he never looks at them and continues to move his leg. When asked to describe the situation, Nick takes a defensive stance and says: "I don't know why I did it; it happened". The behaviours of the family members attract the therapist's attention, since they indicate that participants were involuntary creating a relational context in which Nick embodied the problem: in order to help Nick, the parents and the brother present themselves to the therapists as competent and responsible; paradoxically, this makes Nick feel different from the rest of the family. It becomes clear to the therapist that the family's experience of going through a trial and being assessed by social workers has triggered a defensive reaction, which family members manifest in different ways according to their role. Nick withdraws, whereas the father and the older brother show accountability and rectitude. The therapist acknowledges that the problem brought by the family is difficult and that it is often hard to discuss such private and sensitive matters with strangers; however, she also points out that therapy does not imply evaluation. This is what the therapist says: "I am not a police officer. I care for families and their needs and try to help when people have problems. It seems that in this phase of your family life there is a need that concerns all 4 of you, your relationships, the ways you communicate and get along together. You bravely decided to come here together and look for counselling to try to understand what kind of family you will become after this episode. Everyone should feel free to say what they think and answer to the questions they want. I respect everyone's timing: there might be someone who wants to speak first and others who might want to take more time. Thus, there is no rush ... if I ask a question and 1 of you wants to answer another time, it is absolutely fine! Feel free to answer when it is the best time for you to do that. I am not concerned about that. I think everyone should take their own time".

This intervention has multiple goals: first, the therapist wants to convey the idea that the problem concerned the whole family, not only 1 member, and that coming to therapy was difficult for everybody since it implied taking risks for the sake of their relationships. Also, she acknowledges that everybody is entitled to take time to participate and talk during the therapy session given the difficult issues discussed. The therapist's words have an impact on Sarah and Sean's disclosure: almost at the end of the first session they say that Nick's episode had undermined their confidence as parents. This aspect proves to be crucial for the subsequent sessions since it allows Nick to open up and talk about his worries, while Sam could step down from the role of the "third parent" to get closer and empathize with his brother.

The creation of a Safety context allows clients to show their vulnerabilities, thereby favouring emotional connection [Escudero and Friedlander 2017]. Feeling safe does not necessarily mean "feeling good", but it means readiness to show one's own vulnerabilities to the therapist and other family members.

As underlined by Dee Watts-Jones [2010], the creation of a context in which clients feel safe to explore any issue is also linked to how therapists themselves are comfortable to address explicitly differences and similarities between them and their clients in terms of identities and social positioning associated with power relations and privileges. As a contribution to the construction of a safe context, the author encourages therapists to invite clients in a conversation about the eventual intersection of their social identities that are relevant to the therapeutic relationship (race, ethnicity, gender, social status, age, religion, sexual orientation, etc.). In this way, therapists set the context for these issues to be raised throughout the development of therapy when they become relevant to the meaning-making process and to the quality of the therapeutic relationship.

Emotional connection to the therapist

Emotional Connection to the Therapist refers to clients viewing the therapist as an important person in their life and having a sense that their relationship is based on trust, caring, and concern. Also, it has to do with the feeling that the therapist "is there" for the client and is on the same wavelength [Friedlander *et al.*, 2006]. Emotional connection mainly concerns individual therapies, since it highlights the characteristics of the relationship created between the client and therapist. However, in conjoint therapy it is worth remembering that what happens between 1 family member and the therapist has an impact on family relationships and on the relationship that the other family members have with the therapist. The colleagues who have elaborated SOFTA [Friedlander *et al.* 2006] have pointed out that outside of the therapy sessions, family members discuss how the therapist behaved with themselves and with the others. Clients tend to be more motivated when they realize that the therapist establishes a good connection with family members that are more vulnerable, reluctant to the treatment, or more frightened.

A good emotional connection can be observed when clients verbalize trust in therapists, express interest, and sometimes, affection towards them, even joking with them; in a nutshell, clients feel understood by therapists. Some conditions favour the establishment of a good emotional connection: if clients and the therapist have similar life experiences or backgrounds, values or common worldviews, and similar personalities, it is easier to get along well and establish an emotional connection. Nonetheless, clients' motivation also plays a central role: if clients are highly motivated to start therapy, they will see the treatment as an opportunity to feel better, thus facilitating the creation of a trusting relationship. Therapists can foster emotional connection in different ways: empathizing with clients' suffering; normalizing clients' vulnerabilities; showing interest in clients' story; and sharing their own feelings, personal experiences, and stories to build affiliation and emotional closeness with clients [Friedlander *et al.* 2006]. Therapists should also bear in mind that they should use all this when they feel that the emotional connection is threatened, as illustrated in the case example below.

A therapist is contacted by a young men, Simon, who asks for therapy. After the death of his mother, which occurred a few months earlier, the relationship with his father has deteriorated to the point of having frequent conflicts. Simon appears very motivated to reflect upon his situation, and he wants to overcome these problems to dedicate himself to his own family, since he and his wife have a 3-year-old son and are expecting a second child who will be born in a few months. He says: "for my family, I want to feel better and find a new balance". Simon is aware that the loss of his mother is recent and that his feelings of emptiness, sadness, and despair are normal and appropriate to the situation. However, he is also extremely angry with his father, who has changed from the perfect model of husband, caring for his wife before and during her illness, to a totally different person. Immediately after the wife's death, Simon's father started to date other women; he openly talks about them with Simon and introduces them to their acquaintances. Simon feels that, because of this, the connection with his father is gone, and he wants to distance himself from his father for his shameful behaviours.

In the subsequent sessions, Simon and the therapist explore the loss of the mother. The client provides details about his mother's diagnosis of cancer and the poor prognosis, the agony and the suffering for the months he spent in and out of the hospital caring for her, and his sense of helplessness. After some sessions, the therapist realizes she feels stuck and finds it difficult continuing with Simon; therefore, she decides to ask for a peer supervision.

The therapist's feelings signal problems at the emotional-relational level: she reports that the client's detailed accounts of his mother's illness and death have brought her back to the same situation she experienced 1 year earlier, when she lost her own mother. More specifically, on the one hand, Simon's sad story evoked the therapist's painful emotional memories of her mother's illness; on the other hand, she felt she had to adhere to her professional role, and as a therapist, she should control her emotional reactions and certainly not talk about her own feelings and problems with the client. During the supervision session, 2 contrasting positions emerge, namely: feeling emotionally involved in a situation and taking a "distant" position as required for professional conduct. The therapist fears that these difficulties could undermine the alliance with Simon, especially the emotional connection. The colleagues' feedback focuses on the following issues: can a therapist talk about herself in the therapy session? By definition, in psychotherapy, the focus is on the client; generally, therapists should not talk about their own experiences to show how clients should behave in that particular situation, and they should omit information about their own life whenever they feel that the co-construction of meanings can create a negative relational context for clients (see Chapter 4). Nonetheless, in some situations, such as in Simon's case, therapists' disclosure can be functional to the therapy positive outcome [Roberts 2005]. The colleagues and the therapist reach this conclusion, building upon the items of the SOFTA model used to assess the therapeutic alliance, in particular the dimension of emotional connection. SOFTA validation studies have shown that sharing emotions with clients in a controlled way, strengthens the therapeutic alliance [Carpenter, Escudero and Rivett 2008].

The therapist is relieved by the fact she can share with Simon her emotions in relation to the client narration of his mother's illness. Simon is struck by the therapist's disclosure and takes a listening and reflective position. In turn, the therapist reports that she regained confidence in the relationship with the client and felt that the embarrassment and distance resulting from silencing her emotions dissolved, and an emotional connection was re-established. The therapy ended a few months later when Simon felt he had regained his well-being, had redefined the relationship with his father, and could commit himself to his family that had meanwhile welcomed a baby girl.

This case example clearly shows how emotional connection should not be confined to the initial session; it should instead be nurtured throughout the therapy sessions, to maintain a positive therapeutic alliance. In fact, particularly distressing issues can be addressed only later on in the therapeutic process; therefore, in order to favour changes, emotional connection needs to be monitored at any stage of the therapeutic process.

Shared sense of purpose within the family

Family alliance was originally described by Pinsof [1994] to underline the influence of the relationships that families develop during therapy sessions on the motivation to change, on the actual change, and on the psychotherapeutic outcome. In the SOFTA model [Friedlander *et al.* 2006], the Sense of Shared Purpose measures how much family members invest, together, in the therapy. This dimension refers to how much they perceive they are working in an active and collaborative way to improve their relationships and achieve common goals.

When clients agree on the definition of the problem and are willing to mutually commit to work on what worries them, the therapist is facilitated in conducting the therapy. Generally, if family members realize they cannot solve a problem on their own, they will seek professional advice, having a clear goal shared among family members. If this is the case, they will be able to accept compromise, share jokes, and show sincere interest in others' points of view. Vice versa, therapists may have serious difficulties in conducting the therapy when family members manifest different needs and divergent ideas through disqualification of others' points of view, mutual accusations, and disagreements. These behaviours indicate that the therapist should help clients to see how therapy can benefit everyone. In some cases, families are likely to start a therapy with either a weak shared purpose or a shared purpose that decreases during the sessions. For instance, poorer, more deprived, and multi-stressed families with a chaotic family structure can hardly share a clear definition of the therapeutic goal [Escudero and Friedlander 2017]. Also, the family shared goal can be threatened by the emergence of a difficult topic in front of which family members disagree about how and whether to address it. Furthermore, the success of therapy can undermine the family stability: this happens when the person with the problem starts to change but also when the whole family system is prompted to change. Sometimes, therapists' intervention can also unwittingly affect the shared sense of purpose of the family, as illustrated in the case below.

Claire contacts a family therapist because she worries about her daughter Mary, who is 29. According to Claire, Mary "does not have a purpose in life and never finishes the projects that she starts". Frank, the father, is a physiotherapist and owns a private clinic with his wife, Claire, who is a gynaecologist, and his son, Richard, 35 years old, who works as administrator. Mary is studying to become a physiatrist with the idea of working in the clinic with the rest of the family, but she has attended the School of Medicine for 10 years[2] and is now stuck with the exams. Since the first interview, Claire and Frank have provided different interpretations of the situation. According to the father, Mary is the problem; he says: "Mary continues to say she wants to finish the university; I think she will never do that ... actually, I really do not understand what bothers her". According to the mother, Mary is not the problem; she says: "I do not think Mary is the problem; actually, we are the problem. Both our children are still too dependent on us". Claire underlines that Richard is still living with them, and he is not really interested in expanding his job outside of the family firm. Moreover, she describes him as ambivalent in the relationship with her: sometimes he is a loving son, but other times he is grumpy and choleric. Frank disagrees with his wife: he describes Richard as a skilled professional, very independent and willing to build up his own life outside of the family. Claire adds that their children's problems are somewhat related to their problems as a couple. In particular, she complains because her husband has always been too indulgent with the children, so she has to set the rules, thereby becoming the target of children's anger and discontent. After this statement, Frank gets angry and starts to withdraw from the conversation: he avoids looking at his wife and starts giving vague answers, such as: "I don't think so" and "I don't remember". Claire sits sulky.

The first interview with the couple clearly shows that both parents are concerned for their daughter; however, they have conflicting views. On the one hand, Frank is aware of Mary's problem, but he does not know how to help her; therefore, for him this is the main aim of therapy. Claire concurs with this goal; however, she also introduces the idea that both children have problems that are linked to the couple relationship; therefore, she thinks that therapy should address this issue. The parents' different views about the purpose of the therapy, together with Claire's accusatory attitude towards her husband, and Frank's withdrawal from the conversation, signal that the shared purpose is very weak and the therapeutic alliance is at risk. For this reason, the therapist decides to conclude the first session highlighting the commonalities in the partners' points of view. In particular, she re-addresses the focus of the conversation on Mary's difficulties and suggests the parents to find a moment to talk together with their daughter and share their concerns, while showing openness and acceptance.

After the conversation with Mary about their concerns on finishing the university, the parents report an improvement in Mary's behaviour towards them. However, they continued to be concerned about her future. The therapist asks the parents: "How do you think Mary would respond if you suggested her to work in your clinic, even if she hasn't finished the university?" Frank and Claire consult each other and agree that she might respond positively and that it is worth trying. This reassures the therapist about the creation of a positive alliance among the partners, and about the fact that the focus on helping Mary consolidated the shared sense of purpose within the couple. At the end of the session, they agree that Frank will talk to Mary.

Coming to the third session, Frank appears satisfied since he was able to talk to Mary a couple of days before the session, and their conversation went very well. He refers that he took advantage of Mary's visit to the clinic to talk to her. She seemed comfortable enough to tell him that she had been thinking of leaving medicine and moving to physiotherapy, and she asked her father to let her do some practice in the clinic 1 day a week. According to Frank, after this conversation Mary was relieved. While he describes the conversation with his daughter, Claire is not paying attention; therefore, the therapist decides to involve her:

Therapist:	Claire, did you also notice that Mary was relieved after the conversation with Frank?
Claire:	No, I didn't. I wasn't there, so I didn't notice anything, and he didn't even tell me that he had talked to Mary ... that's how he is ... my husband thinks he is entitled to share nothing about their relationship; he has always been like that.. I haven't noticed anything because I've been completely cut off ... I've been kept out of the information, and I'm very disappointed for that ... Not that I wanted to be present during the meeting ... we had agreed that he would do it. He had to tell me afterwards ... I am his wife ... . Instead, he never tells me anything ... . He doesn't talk ...
Therapist:	Frank, why didn't you tell your wife about your conversation with Mary?
Fank:	I didn't tell her because ... I really don't know why; there's no particular reason ...
Claire (laughing sarcastically):	So, Mary knows it's better not talking to me. Frank has always done that. This shows how our relationship is and has always been!
Therapist:	Do you understand why she felt so disappointed? Did she feel excluded?
Frank:	But she's always ... I don't know ... it's understandable ... yes, maybe ...
Therapist:	She says: "He knew how important this was for me, but ... "
Clear:	Yes, precisely so ... you know ...
Frank:	The normal behaviour would have been for me to call her right after the meeting... and ... explain what happened ... Well, my justification is that I didn't do it ... . this is how I am ...

The spouses keep contrasting positions throughout the session, as they used to do at the beginning of therapy. Claire expresses disappointment by criticizing her husband; in turn, Frank withdraws from the conversation.

How can we explain what happened? While the therapist was exploring Claire's point of view, she unwittingly accepted Claire's definition of the problem, namely the children's problems were related to the couple's problem. In this definition, Frank feels blamed and withdraws. In other words, with the intent of strengthening the alliance, the therapist aligned with Claire, who showed how she felt excluded as wife, thus focusing on the couple's problems. But this had the effect of supporting her point of view against Frank, who had made it clear that he accepted therapy to address Mary's problem, and he was not willing to address the issue of the couple's relationship. This has undermined the parents' shared sense of purpose, thereby lessening the therapeutic alliance with *both of them*. Retrospectively, the therapist should have been aware of this move and should have re-addressed the focus on the shared purpose: Mary's future. This case shows the importance of the therapists being able to maintain an awareness about whom they feel aligned with and why.

Engagement in the therapeutic process

Engagement in the therapeutic process indicates how important clients consider treatment to be. The therapeutic context, in fact, cannot be conceived as a context of application of techniques, prescriptions, and tasks passively received by clients. Their participation is the essential condition for therapy to take place; to participate, a client must feel involved – that is, take therapy seriously and believe that change is possible.

Clients' Engagement in the Therapeutic Process is the most well-known dimension of therapeutic alliance, since it was originally conceptualized by Bordin in the 1970s [Bordin 1979]. Good levels of engagement can be ob-served when clients show specific behaviours, such as: active participation in the definition of the therapy goals by exploring the problems and their possible solutions as well as considering subgoals; completing therapy tasks; acknowl-edging small changes; and reflecting upon the topics emerged in the ther-apeutic conversations [Friedlander *et al.* 2006].

It should be underlined that clients' engagement in the therapeutic process is culturally dependent. Clients from other cultures might have a different conception of what part therapy plays in their well-being or might be con-nected to other sources of healing [for an example, see the case in Davolo and Fruggeri 2016, pp. 117–120]. This is why therapists should be interested in clients' theories of change and the contexts in which these have formed as part of engaging in therapy.

We also want to reiterate that in order to examine the dimension of en-gagement across the therapy sessions, therapists should take into account the differences between individual and conjoint therapy. In individual therapy, clients can decide the topics they want to bring to the therapists' attention, the timing and the strategies they want to use, as well as decide to interrupt therapy if not satisfied. In couple and family therapy the pace of therapy and the commitment to it rely on the level of participation of all members involved. Sometimes, creating a good level of engagement can be very complex and the therapist needs to expressly work on this. The case example reported below illustrates this situation.

Stella contacts a private clinical practitioner since she would like to talk about her relationship with Hillary, her partner, with whom she has been living for 10 years. The woman reports she has been angry towards her partner and doubtful about the continuation of their relationship. In the first interview with the couple, it clearly emerges that Stella and Hillary do not share the same view about starting couple therapy. Stella looks a bit nervous since she "forced" her partner to undertake a therapy; however, she is determined to talk with the therapist about the relationship with Hillary, who on her part is visibly uncomfortable: she sits almost behind her partner and keeps her coat on throughout the session. The 2 women appear very different: Stella is cheerful and sociable, works as a freelance translator, loves travelling, and has a large group of friends. Also, she seems very confident in disclosing feelings and episodes of her private life. Hillary is shy and introverted; she works as a financial consultant and has a passion for swimming. She has few friends and likes her home routines. The couple faced a crisis almost 6 months earlier: Stella told her partner she was tired of fighting because of the conflicts that Hillary had with her family of origin and decided to take a break and move to a common friend's house for 1 month. During that period, Stella felt that Hillary became very dependent on her; this increased Stella's anger towards the partner. Hillary responded that she cared for their couple relationship and that she decided to start therapy to make Stella happy. Nevertheless, during the conversation she expresses her scepticism about the effectiveness of therapy since she believes that: "there is no need to see a therapist to make things work among us". In the first session, the therapist can hardly involve Hillary: she responds to the therapist's questions vaguely ("I do not know", "I haven't thought about that", etc.) or claims she has not heard the questions to the extent that the therapist must repeat the same questions several times. Also, she often looks out of the window and gets easily distracted during the conversation. All the therapist's efforts to engage Hillary are null. The therapist finishes the first session arranging another appointment with both; nonetheless, Stella seems very appreciative and available, whereas Hillary looks hesitant.

In preparation for the second session, the therapist decides that the main goal is Hillary's engagement in the therapy. Hillary's reticent behaviour not only prevented the therapist from exploring the couple's dynamics – the main therapeutic goal – but also threatened Stella's motivation to continue therapy. When a client seems either indifferent or unwilling to participate in the therapy, therapists should focus on this specific aspect with the aim of fostering the alliance with the whole system. Reflecting upon the first session, the therapist realized she insisted on questioning Hillary almost in an investigative way and aligned mainly with Stella's idea that they see a therapist for their couple problem. Therefore, the therapist decides to start the second session rebalancing the alliance. They both come, but the attitude has not changed. Hillary continues to keep her coat on and taps her fingers on the chair. The therapist tells Hillary that she has thought a lot about the first session and that she realized that she had not acknowledged enough how it can be difficult to talk about private issues and share feelings with a stranger. This statement attracts Hillary's attention. Also, the therapist appreciates her effort to come to therapy to please her partner and asks her whether Stella and the therapist could do anything to make her feel comfortable. Appreciating the clients' effort to change – such as the fact of coming to therapy even when there are no observable changes yet – is a key to the creation of a context that favours engagement in the process. In fact, this shows that the therapist understands the clients' effort and respects their time. Additionally, directly asking Hillary to help Stella and the therapist to make her feel comfortable allows Hillary to take a proactive position in the therapeutic relationship and abandon the peripheral and sceptical position she took in the first session. Eventually, Hillary can say she is concerned for not knowing what to expect from both the therapist ("What will we talk about?", "What will the therapist ask?") and Stella ("What will she say about us?"). Hillary's disclosure favoured the creation of a new therapeutic conversation focused on how to talk about the couple's problems without feeling jeopardized. Therefore, this line of conversation allowed both Stella and Hillary to be equally engaged in the therapy process, and to work together for the definition of the therapy goals.

Emotional Connection, Engagement, Shared Purpose, and Safety are crucial dimensions for the development of a good alliance with clients, together with the ability to monitor it throughout the therapeutic process.

The therapeutic alliance is 1 of the components of the relational competency. In the next chapter, we will explore another key component of the relational competency, namely the ability to analyze meanings, identities, and relationships that the therapist and clients co-construct during the therapy. We will describe how this ability will allow therapists to effectively contribute to the construction of transformative contexts.

Notes

1 SOFTA tools can be downloaded for free from this website: http://softa-soatif.com/
2 In Italy, students begin Medical School at the age of 19 after high school, which lasts for 5 years.

References

Beck, M., Friedlander, M.L. and Escudero, V. [2006], *Three perspectives on clients' experiences of the therapeutic alliance: a discovery-oriented investigation*, in Journal of Marital and Family Therapy, 32, pp. 355–368.

Bordin, E. [1979], *The generalizability of the psychoanalytic concept of the working alliance*, in Psychotherapy: Theory, Research and Practice, 16, pp. 252–260.

Carpenter, J., Escudero, V. and Rivett, M. [2008], *Training family therapy students in conceptual and observation skills relating to the therapeutic alliance: an evaluation*, in Journal of Family Therapy, 2008, 30, pp. 411–424.

Davolo, A. and Fruggeri, L. [2016], *A systemic-dialogical perspective for dealing with cultural differences in psychotherapy*, in I. McCarthy e G. Simon, (eds.), *Systemic therapy as transformative practice*, Farnhill UK, Everything is Connected Press, pp. 111–124.

Dee Watts-Jones, T. [2010], *Location of self: opening the door to dialogue on intersectionality in the therapy process*, in Family Process, 49, 3, pp. 405–420.

Escudero, V., Boogmans, E., Loots, G. and Friedlander, M.L. [2012], *Alliance rupture and repair in conjoint family therapy: an exploratory study*, in Psychotherapy, 49, 1, pp. 26–37.

Escudero, V. and Friedlander, M.L. [2017], *Therapeutic alliances with families: empowering clients in challenging cases*, Berlin, Springer.

Escudero, V., Friedlander, M.L., Varela, N. and Abascal, A. [2008], *Observing the therapeutic alliance in family therapy: associations with participants' perceptions and therapeutic outcomes*, in Journal of Family Therapy, 30, pp. 194–214.

Fife, S.T., Whiting, J.B., Bradford, K. and Davis, S. [2014], *The therapeutic pyramid: a common factors synthesis of techniques, alliance, and way of being*, in Journal of Marital and Family Therapy, 40, 1, pp. 20–33.

Friedlander, M.L., Escudero, V. and Heatherington, L. [2006], *Therapeutic alliances in couple and family therapy: an empirically informed guide to practice*, Washington DC, American Psychological Association.

Friedlander, M.L., Wildman, J., Heatherington, L. and Skowron, E.A. [1994], *What we do and don't know about the process of family therapy*, in Journal of Family Psychology, 8, pp. 390–416.

Gottman, J. [1994], *What predicts divorce*, Hillsdale NJ, Erlbaum.

Horvath, A.O. and Bedi, R.P. [2002], *The alliance*, in J.C. Norcross (ed.) *Psychotherapy relationships that work*, New York, Oxford University Press, pp. 37–69.

Horvath, A.O. and Symonds, B.D. [1991], *Relation between working alliance and outcome in psychotherapy: a meta-analysis*, in Journal of Counseling Psychology, 38, pp. 139–149.

Johnson, L.N., Wright, D.W. and Ketring, S.A. [2002], *The therapeutic alliance in home-based family therapy: is it predictive of outcome?*, in Journal of Marital and Family Therapy, 28, pp. 93–102.

Johnson, S.M. and Talitman, E. [1997], *Predictors of success in emotionally focused marital therapy*, in Journal of Marital and Family Therapy, 23, pp. 135–152.

Knobloch-Fedders, L.M., Pinsof, W.M. and Mann, B.J. [2007], *Therapeutic alliance and treatment progress in couple psychotherapy*, in Journal of Marital and Family Therapy, 33, pp. 245–257

Martin, D.J., Garske, J.P. and Davis, M.K. [2000], *Relation of therapeutic alliance with outcome and other variables: a meta-analytic review*, in Journal of Consulting and Clinical Psychology, 68, pp. 438–450.

Pinsof, W.B. [1994], *An integrative systems perspective on the therapeutic alliance: theoretical, clinical, and research implications*, in A.O. Horvath and L.S. Greenberg (eds.), *The working alliance: theory, research, and practice*, New York, Wiley, pp. 173–195.

Pinsof, W.B. [1995], *Integrative problem-centered therapy*, New York, Basic Books.

Pinsof, W.M. and Catherall, D.R. [1986], *The integrative psychotherapy alliance: family, couple and individual therapy scales*, in Journal of Marital and Family Therapy, 12, 2, pp. 137–151.

Quinn, W.H., Dotson, D. and Jordan, K. [1997], *Dimensions of therapeutic alliance and their associations with outcome in family therapy*, in Psychotherapy Research, 7, pp. 429–438.

Roberts, J. [2005], *Transparency and self-disclosure in family therapy: dangers and possibilities*, in Family Process, 44, pp. 45–63.

Sharf, J., Primavera, L.H. and Diener, M.J. [2010], *Dropout and therapeutic alliance: a meta-analysis of adult individual psychotherapy*, in Psychotherapy: Theory, Research, Practice, Training, 47, 4, pp. 637–645.

Strupp, H.H. [1973], *The interpersonal relationship as a vehicle for therapeutic learning*, in Journal of Consulting and Clinical Psychology, 41, 1, pp. 13–15.

Yoo, H., Bartle-Haring, S. and Gangamma, R. [2016], *Predicting premature termination with alliance at sessions 1 and 3: an exploratory study*, in Journal of Family Therapy, 38, 1, pp. 5–17.

4 The construction of transformative interactive contexts

We now explore the therapeutic process, being aware that what we see depends on what we focus on. In fact, a therapeutic intervention can be described from two points of view: the individual one, which concerns how a therapist reflects and acts to help the clients regain a reasonable state of well-being; and the relational one, which concerns the process of joint construction of meanings, relationships, identities, and social realities that emerge from the interaction between therapist and client, while the therapist acts, or has the intention to act, in the clients' interest.

Individual and joint construction processes

A clarification is necessary before we explore this distinction.

In any interpersonal interaction between two or more individuals, two types of psychological processes are co-present and interconnected: the processes of individual construction and the processes of joint construction [Fruggeri 2012]. Individual construction processes are about the way people take part in interactive situations, and therefore refer to the behavioural, emotional, and symbolic individual processes implied. In fact, people act in the interactive situation according to the meanings they attribute (also because of their socio-cultural contexts) to the situation itself, to one's own and others' behaviours, to their emotional responses to the situation, and according to how all of this relates to their purposes. Thus, when placing the emphasis on the processes of individual construction, we might detect feelings, meanings, goals, values, and behaviours of the people involved in the interaction, and observe how all these elements are inter-connected.

However, the processes implied in individual construction, even in their interconnected nature, do not explain the complexity of interactive interpersonal situations. In fact, while the participants in the interaction are engaged in the intertwining of the strategic, symbolic, emotional, and behavioural processes indicated above, they also contribute to shape a joint process, a "dance" through which they negotiate and co-construct meanings, identities, emotions, relationships, roles, and social realities, which, on the one hand, orient individual behaviours, and, on the other hand, are the result of social and interpersonal

DOI: 10.4324/9781003278092-7

interactions. When observing the processes of joint construction, the focus is not how everyone takes part in the interaction, but rather what they do together.

To underline the structuring function of the interactive processes, several communication scholars have explored the "unintended consequences" of interpersonal and social dynamics [for a review, cf. Lannamann 1991]. According to Shotter [1987], unintended consequences are the result of a joint action, not referable to single individuals, but also not caused by external factors. The participants in the interaction have an active role in forming the path of joint action, but the path itself is contingent, and its effects are independent of individuals' intentions. The outcome of a joint action lies beyond the unilateral control of the single participants. Let's consider the following case.

Leah, 24, begins individual therapy because she has been suffering from panic attacks for several months. According to her, the anxiety she is experiencing is a response to work stress. Leah has been working for a couple of years in her paternal uncle's engineering firm, but she does not like it. Her uncle is a difficult person, who has had problems with depression and whom she finds hyper-controlling; furthermore, he does not pay her adequately. A few months earlier, she had received an offer for a part-time job at another firm; it was an opportunity that she would have liked to take to gradually decrease her commitment to the family enterprise. However, her uncle and father, together, prevented her from doing so. The divergence of views led to serious quarrels, which put Leah in a state of deep anxiety. The therapist begins to explore the family relationships and the dynamics involved in such a rigidly conflictual and painful situation.

Leah lives with her mother; her father; one brother, Robert, aged 30; and two sisters, Mila, aged 27, and Maya, aged 12. The relationship between Leah and her father has never been good, but relations are also tense between the father and mother, who "married because they had to, but they have never got along well". Leah claims she does not expect anything from her father; she is instead afraid of him because he has always been quite aggressive: she fears that he could take revenge on her mother if she opposes him. Recently, Leah wanted to live with her boyfriend, but she didn't want to leave her mother, who repeatedly suggested moving into an apartment with her and the youngest daughter, Maya, thus leaving the other members of the family. Leah is the mother's favourite, and the bond between them is very strong: they comfort each other about their personal concerns (the mother's marital dissatisfaction and Leah's discontent at work). The older brother is not interested in family matters and is "always locked in his room"; he refuses to help around the house and just doesn't care about the other family members. Mila, the older sister, is very involved in the relationship with her boyfriend and is waiting for him to finish law school to start living together; she has detached herself from the mother and sometimes sides with the father. Maya, the youngest, is on the mother's side and hardly talks to the father.

As therapy goes on, Leah feels more and more "trapped" in all areas of her personal life: she cannot decide about her job because she fears this would trigger an unbearable conflict with her father, which in turn could negatively affect her mother; but she cannot decide to leave home either because this would mean "abandoning" her mother, who relies on her to be rescued from her unhappy marriage. To help Leah identify possible resources that could sustain her in stepping out of this stuck situation, and considering the brother's unavailability, the therapist suggests inviting Mila to the session. Leah agrees because she thinks her sister could be supportive. The meeting begins with talking about Leah's unhappiness: Mila had not realized that her sister was in such pain and shows an empathic response that reassures Leah. When it comes to the description of the family dynamics, however, Mila's attitude changes. Faced with the exploration of different points of view on the relational impasse in which Leah finds herself, Mila withdraws and says she does not want to interfere in the relationship between her mom and dad. She argues that Leah must learn how to cope with her own anxiety and should talk to her father without worrying about the consequences.

By inviting Mila, the therapist intended to create a relational context in which Leah could begin to consider alternatives to her situation with the support of her sister. On the contrary, the meeting of the 2 sisters with the therapist turned out to be a context in which the premise according to which Leah is the only one who cares for the mother was reconfirmed. Mila was available to comfort her sister as an outsider, but not to be considered part of the solution to her problem. After this session, Leah interrupted the therapy, sending the therapist a letter in which she wrote "thank you for the great help you have given me, but the situation at home has got worse. I think my sister does not understand me at all, and I don't feel like continuing the therapy anymore".

When inviting Mila to the session, the therapist asked for Leah's opinion, but wasn't as careful to consider Mila's point of view or to evaluate the effects that her action in the context of the relationship with her client (support Leah in taking an independent stance) could have in the context of the relationships her client had with other family members (the effect of Leah becoming independent on her sister's plans). The therapist acted without considering that a different positioning of Leah in the family context would have also entailed a change in Mila's positioning; Mila, in turn, immediately withdrew, leaving Leah in the uncomfortable position of being the "only pivot" of the family, thus undoing the efficacy of the therapeutic intervention (unintended consequence). How could the therapist have addressed this and repositioned herself within the session by observing joint construction, that is, what they were construing in terms of meanings of identities and relationships? The therapist would have realized that Mila was probably feeling put in the position of being responsible for Leah's life; the therapist would then have changed the direction of the conversation: instead of exploring the family relationships, the therapist would have explored with both Mila and Leah the impact of Leah's autonomy on family relationships and on the individual development of family members. This would have offered the therapist the possibility of welcoming Mila's concerns and reassuring both Mila and Leah that Leah's well-being wasn't pursued at the expense of anyone else.

Individual and relational levels in psychotherapy

The distinction between the process of individual construction and the process of joint construction is useful because it helps to define the individual level and the relational level through which to analyze therapeutic interventions [Fruggeri 2002; 2012]. These are 2 different views that highlight different protagonists, mechanisms, devices, structures, and socio-psychological processes.

At the individual level, we focus on the practitioners, their thoughts, intentions, decisions, language, goals, descriptions, theoretical ideas, models, prejudices, values, ideologies, and actions; and on how all these elements connect with each other in a pattern that can be defined as "the way in which the professional participates in the interaction with client". Strategizing [Tomm 1987], described in Chapter 1, is an expression of the individual level of the therapeutic process, as it refers to the questions that therapists ask themselves during interviews with clients, to which they respond based on their specific professional training, personal history, and relational and social experiences. Another expression of the individual level is the decision that the therapist makes, step by step, about how much of the inner dialogue that resonates in response to clients' response, should be communicated and in what ways [Rober 2011]. The level of individual analysis therefore highlights the recursiveness between the theoretical framework, experience, attribution of meaning, actions, and emotional and relational responses of a therapist.

Indeed, professionals make sense of what is happening according to a theoretical model, to their personal professional experiences, their social positioning, as well as to their responses in the relational situation; and they make decisions about what to do according to this understanding.

The focus on the individual level of the intervention evokes the therapist's technical competency, that is, the competency based on the knowledge of procedures, theories, and methodologies, and the ability to apply and use them in connection with specific people, situations, events, and contexts with which professionals deal (see Chapters 1 and 2). It is a skill that develops from being trained in a specific therapeutic model (which could refer to practices ranging from prescriptive-strategic to collaborative), and grows through clinical practice, as well as through experience, supervision, self-awareness paths, reading, and participation in conferences and seminars.

However, practitioners aren't the only ones involved in the situation. Clients, in turn, participate in the interaction starting from their own premises, which are not formal theoretical models, but implicit theories rooted in their belonging to interpersonal, social, and cultural systems. Based on these premises, they give meaning to what happens and, consequently, act. During a conference on group dynamics of schizophrenia, Gregory Bateson made the following comment: "In this conference we have discussed various ways of interacting with patients, describing what we do and what our strategy seems to us to be. It would have been more difficult to describe our actions from the patients' point of view" [1972, p. 230]. Clients, in fact, do not respond to the interventions of professionals based on the intentions or feelings of professionals, but based on their interpretation and responses to what the professionals do. Clients, too, continually question themselves during the interview with the therapist: What is the most useful information to give? What does the therapist think? What understanding has the therapist made of the situation or of the people involved? Clients might also have questions about the therapists' personal life and their cultural belonging. The answers clients give to these questions do not depend on the psychotherapist's theoretical model or viewpoint, but on their own assumptions, their past experiences, their prejudices and ideologies, and their history as human and socio-cultural beings (see Box 4.1).

Box 4.1   Clients' comments about their therapies

It is not uncommon for therapists to encounter clients who have abandoned previous therapies because they have been disappointed in them. In this regard, clients' comments about the reasons for their dissatisfaction are interesting and revealing. We report some of them.

"The doctor wanted at all costs that we change the relationships in our family ... My father had to be more present, and my mother had to find some interests outside the house in order not to be on us children all the time ... he gave us these tasks that we just couldn't do. He insisted, but the only result was that a new problem was added to my problem: my parents began to feel guilty" [a client's comment reported in Cingolani 1995, pp. 115–116].

This reflection is echoed by the comments of a father, collected by one of the authors: "It seemed like it was our fault, as if I, as father, and she, as mother, were unable to raise our children. It seemed that the cause of Nadia's problems was that she [the wife] and I don't go out together" [Personal communication].

Every family therapist may recognize behind these words of mistrust and frustration, the therapist's attempt to apply basic principles of structural family therapy or to promote a reorganization of relationships in such a way that the redefinition of the couple relationship (parental and marital) could favour the autonomous development of children. The therapists in question have certainly operated starting from the best intentions, suggested by their models. In this case, we cannot speak of the therapists' incompetence since they acted according to the principles of their technical model, principles that have probably worked in many other cases. However, they were not effective in those mentioned above. The implicit suggestions, the reflections proposed, and the comments made by the therapists for therapeutic purposes, have been understood, felt, and experienced by the members of these families, as criticisms, blame, and undue requests.

In the following client's comment, we can recognize another type of therapist who does not give advice, prescriptions, or evaluations; he does not propose a point of view to the family. He instead promotes dialogue between family members so that they reflect to let emerge a new vision from the circularity of points of view that can help family members find new solutions. However, the result is similar.

"We had high expectations in that therapy, and at the beginning, things seemed to be going well: everyone liked the doctor. He told us that he should have a picture of the situation first. But then it became a never-ending picture … He made us talk, talk, talk … We were willing to do anything to change. But we hardly talked about Larry's problems at all … about the past, rather. But Larry was getting worse. We were expecting directions on what to do. We asked him questions, but the doctor told us to ask those questions to each other. He, on the other hand, did nothing but question us. Every so often he tried to make us understand that there was something positive in our situation, and that there wasn't much to change. We were beginning to feel … I don't want to say cheated, but certainly not helped" [a client's comment reported in Cingolani 1995, p. 117].

Also in this case, as in the previous one, we cannot speak of technical errors on the part of the therapist; the therapist's actions produced an effect not in accordance with his intentions, but with how the clients, based on their experiences, expectations, and goals, made sense of those actions.

However, the literature documents that the diversity of points of view and interpretations between the therapist and clients can also be found in the therapeutic process with positive outcomes. This is a story collected by Friedlander, Escudero and Heatherington [2006, p. 9].

"A colleague of ours posed this question to one of his clients as their therapeutic work was coming to an end. The therapist had been treating her for nearly 2 years; she had made significant improvement. Thinking the information might be helpful in his work with future clients, he asked her during their last appointment 'What was it about the therapy that was helpful to you?' 'Do you remember the time the bumblebee flew in the window?' she countered. 'Yes', he replied with considerable embarrassment. He was both allergic to and deadly afraid of bees, and her question brought back a vivid image of cowering under the desk while his client chased the bee out of the window. 'That was the turning point for me' she continued 'because until that time I saw that you as a perfect person, but distant and unapproachable. I didn't trust that you could really help or understand me. But when I saw that you had fears and flaws too, that's when I decided I could relate. I opened up. After that, I began to really work in our sessions. It all started to fall into place'".

This story is a nice example of how unpredictable the clients' judgement of the therapists' actions can be. On the other hand, empirical research confirms how the explanations that clients give about the effectiveness of the treatment are different from those of therapists [Hunsley *et al.* 1999; Helmeke and Sprenkle 2000].

The above vignettes illustrate how clients participate in the therapeutic process starting from their own premises and therefore do not respond to the interventions of professionals based on the intentions of professionals but based on the interpretation they give of what professionals do. The recognition of "the unique otherness of the other" is both a scientific and an ethical issue for therapists [Shotter 2010; 2015]. This is the reason why it is necessary to understand the dance that takes shape from the encounter of the therapist's and the client's different perspectives.

While practitioners and clients are engaged in their respective individual processes of construction, they also participate in a cooperative dance, in a joint action through which they negotiate and co-construct their identities, what they are doing together, the situation in which they are involved, their relationship, and their social status and positioning. As underlined by Linell [2009], although a word or a sign gains its meaning from the past and is directed towards a future answer, its actual meaning is created in the encounter in situ. The analysis of this level of the therapeutic intervention does not concern the ideas, actions, objectives, and expectations of professionals, nor the ideas, actions, goals, and expectations of clients. At this level, analysis implies a *relational competency* that enables therapists to describe the joint action of practitioner and client, and the meanings that are generated through it.

In this chapter, we focus on the construction of personal and interpersonal realities, without forgetting that the therapies are meeting places where social realities such as power relationships and socio and cultural identities are also negotiated [Daniel 2012]. We don't want to undermine the recursive relationship between interpersonal, personal, and social experiences [Burnham 2012]; yet, exploring them separately, even if it might be an artificial distinction, allows focusing on the complexity of each level. We will address and develop the social issues in Part III and IV of the book, where we will discuss the social awareness of therapists, the recursiveness of personal, interpersonal, social, and cultural experiences and their implications in the therapeutic process. Here, we want to stress the importance for therapists to be aware of when they operate according to a technical competency or a relational one. From this perspective, in their internal dialogue, therapists can ask themselves questions to which they answer according to their own experience, resonance, and knowledge, or they can ask themselves questions to which they answer according to the analysis of the therapeutic process that they shape together with clients. For example, knowing the importance of establishing a good emotional connection with the client, therapists can ask themself what action, according to theory, should be taken to promote this important dimension of the alliance, thus expressing a technical competency; or therapists can ask themself about the quality of the relationship they are building with that specific client and, starting from this observation, decide what is appropriate to do in order to establish an emotional connection, thus exercising relational competency.

Relational competency is a second-order competency in that it consists of the ability to observe and understand what the therapist and client construct together. The technical competency of family therapists, for example, might guide them to invite the whole family for a session; relational competency could instead induce the therapist to invite only the person who manifests the problem in the family, or only the parents of the person who manifests the symptoms, if it emerges from the analysis of the therapeutic relational context that the coexistence of the parents and children constitutes a context in which the children cannot position themself independently from the parents, or as a context that prevents the parents from addressing issues related to the couple's relationship that appear central to the dynamics underlying individual and family discomfort.

As to the distinction between technical and relational competency, Roy-Chowdhury [2006] proposes an interesting comparison between a therapist who, to remain faithful to her non-directive approach, ends up not welcoming a client who seeks and asks for advice, and a therapist who, to keep the dialogue with the client open, accepts a position of expert who gives advice, thus contributing to build a relational context in which the client feels respected and competent. Relational competency leads practitioners to raise the question suggested by Gregory Bateson: "How do we qualify our communication to the patients, so that the experience which they receive will be therapeutic?" [1972, p. 231].

Psychotherapy as a context for the development of positive identities

Studies on extracts of family discourse taken from everyday life and from therapy sessions have documented that family hierarchy, identities, roles, and psychological states are constructed and deconstructed through conversational strategies [Ervin-Tripp, O'Connor and Rosenberg 1984; Ochs and Taylor 1996; Aronsson and Cederborg 1994; Tannen 2007; Aronsson and Cekaite 2011]. In other words, the discourse defines the positions that individuals take in the interaction [Harré *et al.* 2009]. Thus, we can say that different types of information, relationships, and identities emerge in different conversational contexts. That is why therapists wonder how the context influences the kind of talk and the information being created [Simon 2016]. From this point of view, the analysis of the conversation between the therapist and client is a way to explore the relational level of psychotherapy, to analyze the therapeutic dance, and to point out the meanings that the therapist and clients construct together.

And it is precisely the analysis of the conversational context that allowed the systemic family therapist of the following case[1] to abandon the exploration of family relationships, and to concentrate on issues of an individual nature, when the context of the conversation about relationships emerged as an unhelpful context to build positive identities of all the participants in the interaction [Fruggeri 2012].

The Panni family asks for therapy because of the discomfort shown by their 17-year-old son Fredrick, a brilliant student at the Classical Lyceum, who has, however, been refusing to go to school for months; he only goes out in the evening and only when accompanied by his mother, towards whom, however, he behaves aggressively. When the mother calls asking for therapy, she says, among other information that Fredrick is afraid of being called "faggot" by his schoolmates. The parents recently consulted a psychologist, who referred them to a Family Therapy Institute. Fredrick refuses to attend sessions, which are then conducted only with the parents.

The Panni family lives in a small village in the countryside. The father, Ivan, is a worker in a factory that makes tiles; the mother, Martha, is a housewife. The therapist, as she usually does, leaves the "symptoms" aside for a while (to avoid blaming discourses) and starts exploring the family relationship in order eventually to address the problematic issues within a relational context. From the information gathered, the mother seemed central to the situation both positively (Fredrick wants to go out only with her) and negatively (Fredrick is aggressive only towards her). For this reason, the therapist decides to explore and thus bring out the relationship of Fredrick with his father. The therapist soon realizes that in exploring the father–son relationship tensions emerge between the parents (See Extract 1)

Extract 1

Ter: So, when you and your son are together, he tells you …
Ivan: Yes, many things
Ter: Does he talk about himself?
Ivan: No, not about himself. He hides certain things. That's the way he is.
Ter: Does he talk about his wishes?
Ivan: Yes, his wish is to work as a model in the fashion field, but I say …
Marta: When does he talk to you? I never heard.
Ivan: Yes, he does … . the other day, for example …

Ter:	Ms. Panni, maybe occasionally your son and your husband talk to each other when you are not around.
Ivan:	Exactly!
Marta:	I am not sure!

... ...

Ivan:	I tell Fredrik that he has to behave well. At home we have rules that he needs to respect. He says I must study; leave me alone. He always has some excuse.
Ter:	Does he have excuses for not spending time with you?
Ivan:	I know, I know!!
Ter:	And what explanation do you have?
Ivan:	I think that ... .
Marta:	We are not a perfect couple.
Ivan:	But no, we are a couple like many others. When you work ...
Marta:	Don't bother me about work; everyone in the world works.

... ...

Ter (to father):	Let's go back to the question I asked you. What is your explanation for Fredrik's problems?
Ivan:	I am not very educated. I only have the 5th grade, so I don't know.
Marta:	You know nothing!!!
Ivan:	It could be, but I decided to work, and I like my work and I am happy of my choice. I always say this to Fredrik.
Ter:	What future do you imagine for your son?
Ivan:	I don't know
Ter:	What would you like him to do?
Ivan:	I'd like him to become a good worker!
Marta:	What??? You don't know what you say! A worker??? He is studying for the University.

Unexpectedly for the therapist, the exploration of father–son relationship reveals a context of conversation in which all the persons involved appear to be uncomfortable: the more the therapist, hoping to give recognition to father's position, asks questions about the father and son relationship, the more the mother blames the father who, in turn, takes up a defensive position, thus undoing the therapist's attempts to support his paternal role.

These are the cases when it is not a matter of asking the right or wrong question; it is not a matter of formulating a more or less creative hypothesis either. This is the case when the therapist needs to develop a relational competency, that is, to take a second-order position and observe what the interactive context produces in terms of individual positions and identities. Having taken this perspective, it clearly appeared to the therapist that "talking about father–son relationship" was a context in which participants appeared to feel inadequate; it was then necessary to change the very context of the interview to change the direction of the session.

If, as we wrote above, discourse defines the position of the persons, a change in the position of a participant triggers a change of the conversational context, thus opening the space for different roles to emerge [Jones 2003; Harré *et al.* 2009]. Following this consideration, the therapist decides to abandon the exploration of relationships and chooses to explore the behaviours of Fredrick that worry his parents to position herself differently, and in so doing, to move away from a context that allowed only for negative identities of everyone involved (see Extract 2).

Extract 2

Ter: Ms. Panni, when you called asking for therapy, you said that Fredrik has the great fear to be called "faggot"?

Marta: Yes

Ter: Who thinks he is gay?

Marta: At the beginning I thought he was.

Ter: Since when?

Marta: When I saw that he didn't go out, he was a bit feminine, he was so attached to me, also Dr. Rose said he needed to get closer to his father. At that time, I was afraid he was …

Ter: And now?

Marta: No

Ter: (to Father) And you

Ivan: No!

Marta: He never did … . he never thought he was!

… ..

Ter: (to mother) Do you still have this doubt?

Marta: No, not now. At that time, I was afraid, not that I knew, I was afraid

Ter: And do you think that Fredrik has the doubt that you still have the doubt?

Marta: I don't know.

Ivan: Maybe yes.

Ter: Is it possible that when you express disagreement about his project of becoming a model, he feels you express disappointment about him being gay?

Marta: I never thought about this, but it could be.

Ter:	With whom would Fredrik talk if he decided to talk about this topic?
Ivan:	I think with his mother. But I also think that he might have the courage to tell me, too. Even if with his mother it would be different
Ter:	You know, there is a thing that I can't explain to myself! I see you very accepting and benevolent. So, one would expect that a son would also feel safe to talk about this, but Fredrik doesn't feel safe. He fears the word can be said!! If he were gay and would like to talk …
Marta:	I would accept him as he is.
Ivan:	Whatever … . He will always be my son.

In the new context of conversation, all participants emerge as competent and connected. Talking about Fredrick's fears has turned out to be a context of conversation within which feelings, emotions, and healing words could be expressed. In other therapies with other families with different histories, the context of exploring relationships may be helpful in building positive identities, new meanings, and enlightening connections. For this family, such a conversational context proved useless, if not dangerous, for the relationships and identities of all involved, including the therapist. On the other hand, the kind of conversation that has emerged as useful for Marta and Ivan Panni could constitute, for other families, an occasion for mutual accusations. Choosing when it is the case to activate one or the other type of conversational context is not an a priori. It is a decision that can only be taken by analyzing the interactive process as it unfolds; that is, it can only be taken by implementing relational competency, which, as we said, helps therapists to move from the level of technical content, to observe and understand the contingent process of construction of meanings in which they participate together with their clients.

Psychotherapy as "secure base"

As discussed in the previous paragraph, the issue of positive identity is central to a psychotherapeutic process, since the therapist's responsibility is not only to help clients, but also to build transformative relational contexts, which generate clients' positive self-image, that is, contexts within which clients feel valued and feel in charge of their life. In Chapter 3, we discussed the importance of developing a good therapeutic alliance between the therapist and clients. Positive identity and good relationship are two very important factors for the success of a therapy. Nevertheless, in this regard, it is important to underline that the therapeutic relationship cannot be generative if it creates addiction, that is, if people have the need to maintain the therapeutic relationship to continue to feel well. The client's dependence is an unintended consequence that is visible to therapists only if they analyze the relationship they are building with clients. Being a welcoming context, psychotherapy risks creating addiction if it is not connoted as a "secure base" [Byng-Hall 1995], that is, as a starting point for the exploration of other significant relationships. Let's see the following case.

James is a 29-year-old young man who asks for therapy following the advice of the head of the educational community where he has been working as an educator for 1 year. James is Paul and Elisabeth's only child; he lived with his parents and his maternal grandfather until 6 months ago, when he started living with his girlfriend, Eleonor (with whom he has been engaged for 10 years), at her house, where her mother and brother also live.

James describes himself as a determined person with a "normal" life, who at a certain point found himself having to deal with problems that he was not aware of. He recently experienced moments of fragility and emptiness related to his difficulty in coping with the stories of the disadvantaged children he meets in his work.

During the therapeutic encounters, James appears very involved; he attends the sessions with commitment and regularity every 2 weeks for about 1 year. The past story he tells about himself is a successful one; he has always been perfect in all fields of his life: excellent academic achievements, lots of friends, a steady girlfriend since high school, politically and socially involved. He has always been guided by a great sense of duty and responsibility. After high school, though, James has begun to feel a growing sense of bewilderment: old friends have taken different roads; the academic and professional perspectives have become less and less clear (what do I want to do when I grow up?); the relationship with his girlfriend began to oscillate between alternate periods of detachment and rejoining; the religious and political involvement became more and more disappointing, and less and less engaging; finally, he began to feel his family's concern for his uncertain life choices.

The therapy focuses on how to deal with his uncertainties, on the differences between what "must be done" and what he wishes to do. After a year, James appears more satisfied with his daily life, work, and life choices. At this point, the therapist underlines the goals achieved and proposes to set the next meeting after the summer (after a 2-month break). James agrees with both the goals achieved and the date of the next session.

In September, when he returns to therapy, he describes a negative scenario. During the summer months, he has experienced several moments of anxiety and panic related to work, but not only that; he says he worries about his situation. He refers to 2 episodes of the past that had not emerged previously, but which he feels the need to explore, and asks to resume the therapeutic encounters regularly and systematically.

The therapist is uncertain about how to explain this new and unexpected scenario. Was the 2-month interval a mistake? Should the therapist have proposed a shorter break? Did the therapist make a wrong evaluation with respect to the goals achieved to that point? These are all legitimate questions inspired by technical competence – questions, though, whose answers bring the process back in a sort of "let's start again with the right foot", as if processes could go back and forth in time!

The therapist considers instead implementing her relational competency and exploring the meaning of James's request in the context of the co-construction process that took place in their relationship. Psychotherapy is a creative process in which the meanings of the client and those of the therapist come into contact, producing new meanings, different from the initial ones [Rober 2005]. Others are then the questions that can be asked from this point of view: What meanings did James and the therapist build together in their relationship? What *meaning did the 2-month interval take in the relational context constructed by James and the therapist during their interaction?* This kind of questions emerges from the implementation of a relational competency.

The questions that therapists can raise from a technical point of view versus a relational point of view are different in form: they are not different questions but different *types* of questions. Technical competency suggests questions that, starting from the client's feedback, wonder about the accuracy of the therapist's intervention. Relational competency invites reflection on the context of meaning that the therapist and client have constructed together and on how this has become the context of meanings of the subsequent actions taken by the therapist and client.

Taking a relational perspective, the therapist considers the possibility that the positive evolution of therapy has produced both James's greater well-being and his fear of emancipation from therapy that the greater well-being would entail. The therapist reflects on the possibility that James may have been frightened by the idea of losing the therapeutic relationship and of having to "stand on his own feet". In this respect, the new problematic issues he reported were feeding the maintenance of the therapeutic relationship. These considerations also help the therapist to focus on how much James's life has become, especially in recent years, short on meaningful relationships and, therefore, how much the therapeutic relationship may have become a comfortable and safe relational context, a substitute for the relationships in his daily life. From this point of view, the possibility emerges that the therapy has produced an improvement in the client's life, but also a dependence on the therapy, thus leading to the paradox that to maintain the relationship with the therapist, the client must not improve. The notion of secure base [Byng-Hall 1995] is inspiring and helpful to overcome this paradox, because, as we said, it allows one to think of therapy as a safe and reassuring space, which is however a starting point for the exploration of other significant relationships.

Beginning from these considerations, as in the previous case, the therapist decides to position herself differently in the process. She agrees to continue therapy as requested by James, who in fact seems to be reassured, but the work that the therapist now suggests is different: following her reflections, she asks

James if he would like Eleanor, his girlfriend, to attend their meetings. The therapist sees James's relationship with Eleanor as a potential resource, in fact, the only significant relationship he seems to have now. James approves the idea. He talks to Eleanor, and both agree to attend the sessions together. The therapy is oriented to themes shared by the couple: their mutual feelings, their future goals, the importance of making roots, planning a housing situation independent of their families of origin, and how Eleanor could help James in the process of becoming more emotionally independent from his family. Eleanor appears very reassuring to James, who can see how important he is for her as he is, with strengths and weaknesses, thus dismantling the idea that he has always had of being loved only if "perfect". On the other hand, Eleanor can see how important she is for James. Therapy takes on a new form. After a few months, the therapist can also prepare her separation from James, who now feels safe in another significant relationship, the one with Eleonora, with whom he will plan their future life.

Intertwining relational and technical competencies

Technical and relational competencies are not mutually exclusive. Indeed, they offer a double vision: one oriented by the theoretical model or by the responses of the therapist to the situation, the other by the analysis of the therapeutic process as it unfolds and takes shape.

From this point of view, the questions that therapists might ask themself in their inner dialogue about the most appropriate issues to raise, the most appropriate interpretation to make, and the most useful comments to express, do not find an answer only in the technical model or in the therapist's intuition or bodily responses. The criterion for deciding if an idea is valid, if an opinion can be accepted, or if a proposal could be rejected must also be sought in the meanings emerging from the interaction between the therapist and clients.

The following case is an example of how the therapist reorients the therapeutic process after reflecting on how the type of story she had participated in building with her clients prevented her from addressing other emotionally difficult issues.

Sonia and Philip ask for therapy due to a crisis in their couple relationship. They are both 42 years old, have been a couple for 15 years, and have been living together for 12. They have a 6-year-old daughter who is in first grade. They describe their life as satisfying and comfortable: he is a pharmacist, and she is an architect.

They trace their problems back to about a year earlier, when during a discussion which they now both define as senseless, Philip pushed Sonia hard, causing her to fall and develop very strong back pain, which still sporadically reoccurs, reminding her of the violent episode.

There have been no other events of this nature, either before or after. Philip says he is frightened, he does not understand the reason for his gesture, and he has become depressed ever since. Sonia radically changed her idea of him. She began to perceive him as disconnected and, at times, even "mean". Both describe their life as marked by before and after the episode: before there is a past characterized by a normal, happy, and evolving situation; after there is a present characterized by silence, distance, and an everyday life exclusively focused on the care of their child. Sonia says she has tried several times to leave what happened behind without ever succeeding; she perceives her partner as distant and interested only in their daughter, with whom he has an excellent relationship, from which however she feels excluded. Philip says he is very sorry for what happened and wants to go on and recreate the emotional climate preceding the fateful event. The psychotherapist is the first person to whom they tell the episode that struck them so much. For this reason, she leaves room in their conversations for the description of what happened, the meanings attributed, and the immediate and subsequent emotional reactions.

The exploration of relationships with their respective families of origin does not give any significant information: Philip's parents live far away, whereas Sonia's parents live in the same city and are a resource for the whole family. Philip has an excellent relationship of affection and esteem with his in-laws to the point that, Sonia claims, his behaviour during their argument would be inconceivable, as well as incomprehensible, to them.

Among the various information, they report that a year before her pregnancy, Sonia discovered that she has a rare degenerative disease. Almost at the same time, Philip discovered that he is a carrier of a pathology from which his mother suffers. Shortly after this news, Sonia became pregnant, and they strengthened their relationship, promising everlasting mutual support. Since then, Philip's clinical situation has remained stable and does not affect his daily life, whereas for Sonia, in recent years, a gradual worsening of the clinical picture has begun forcing her to a series of limitations such as not being able to drive a car. Only their families know of the diseases, no one else. Recently Sonia has been compelled to communicate it at her workplace in order to receive the benefits she is entitled to have because of her pathology. In talking about their health situation, they tend to be brief, rapidly changing topic of conversation. The therapist also abandons the subject of the physical pathologies to focus on the couple relational issues, since they report the persistence of their mutual misunderstandings. The therapist decides to explore the theme of separation: Sonia says she thought about it and talked about it to Philip, but both exclude it as a solution; they want instead to engage in couple therapy to overcome their discomfort.

A few meetings are dedicated to "who are you for me", "who am I for you", how much Sonia thinks she can forgive Philip, what he feels he can do to be forgiven, and if there can be a space for future planning for the couple after the incident. They continue to express a deep nostalgia for how beautiful their life used to be and a deep regret since it cannot be any longer like it was.

The therapist begins to feel helpless and wonders about what she and the couple are constructing together. The story they are telling is a story of regret, disappointment, and sadness. The therapist feels unable to help them to consider another point of view. Speaking of the case in a peer-to-peer supervision, the therapist is invited to take a second-order position. Starting with the question "what have we built together?" the psychotherapist reviews the process and the information that has emerged; then it becomes clear that what they have built together is collusion in avoiding the issue of the physical diseases. Reflecting on this aspect, the therapist shares with her colleagues that indeed she feels uncomfortable in the face of clients' discomfort in talking about their diseases, and she realizes that she accepted the clients' feedback to skip the topic and move on to explore other issues. The motto "Let's pretend that there are no diseases" that governs Philip and Sonia's daily life was also regulating the therapeutic context. These considerations led to new questions: How much did Sonia and Philip elaborate the limitations and risks that their pathologies entail? How much have they been able to talk about the anger and worries connected to their health status? How much have these feelings over time undermined their relationship to the point of developing reciprocal aggressive behaviours and feelings? What anxieties affect the future? What are the concerns for their daughter: will Philip have passed on his pathology to her? How can Philip and Sonia keep the mutual support agreement stipulated after their respective diagnoses, if each of them is committed to containing their own distress? The emotional charge of these issues, which is also shared by the therapist, suggests that after all it is easier to cope with the violent episode than with the diagnosed pathologies. In this sense, the violent episode became protective, it created a barrier between the two of them, preventing them from facing something even more painful. This reflection convinces the therapist to redefine the goal of therapy from repairing an unpleasant episode to the elaboration of a shared distress.

Communication on this pain can no longer be postponed, but the question is "How can the therapist avoid forcing their feelings, with the risk of losing the therapeutic alliance?" Keeping in mind Bateson's question reported above ("How do we qualify our communication to the patients so that the experience that they receive will be therapeutic?"), the therapist decides to talk about the discomfort in addressing a topic so full of suffering and takes up the taboo theme in this way: "In the course of our meetings, various questions emerged, and we talked about many issues of your past, present, and future life. I realized, however, that there is one issue that I have not been able to explore with you, and I wondered why. I refer to your illnesses … when we tried to talk about it, almost immediately we moved on to other topics. Why do you think we did that? For my part, I feel that it was difficult because it is a subject full of unknowns and pain. How is it for you to talk about it?" With this intervention, the therapist shifts the focus from diseases to the difficulty in talking about them, taking the responsibility upon herself, letting them join eventually, without pushing them to face what they couldn't yet face. She triggered a process of *relational reflexivity* with the clients, which enabled them to make a choice as to whether to discuss the sensitive topic or not [Burnham 2005]. Starting from this conversation, a new space for dialogue opens; both Sonia and Philip agree about feeling distressed and of having "learned" over the years to ignore it for fear of "seeing" what could happen. Sonia admits she thinks about it a lot, whereas Philip says he doesn't think about it at all. At this point, their fears for the future emerge; these mainly concern their daughter, but also themselves. A space for dialogue and expression of their emotions and their anxieties begins; together with the communication emerges the desire for a greater sharing of these issues by the couple. Therapy takes up a new generative path.

As can be seen from this case, relational competency allows for a constant understanding of the interactive process undertaken with clients, to monitor the relational process and to "adjust" one's action to contribute to the construction of interactive situations in which clients can express their resources and find answers to their needs.

This case shows how technical competency and relational competency are interconnected, offering a complex vision of the therapeutic process, a double vision as Bateson defines it, a vision that makes use of information deriving from different types of sources [Bateson 1979]. In the therapeutic field, it means combining observation of the client's relationships with that of the relationship between the therapist and client [Fruggeri 1998].

Technical competency and relational competency are in dialogue with each other in such a way that relational competency, offering a different vision of the therapeutic process, provides ideas for creative and generative technical interventions. The case described above shows how the analysis of the process of construction produced by the interaction between the therapist and clients has given ideas for reorienting the therapist's technical interventions by introducing, in an acceptable way for the clients, the most difficult and most significant issues.

The question that is often raised as to whether therapy should be considered a science or an art reveals a dualistic approach that opposes expertise to creativity, technique to relationship, and rigor to imagination. Instead, the perspective we have illustrated proposes combining these dichotomies. In fact, it implies that therpists exercize their professional competency with creativity, that they apply technical models based on the analysis of the relational interactive process that takes shape during therapy. It is a perspective that implies therapists who, to best express the resources of their technical approach, take care first to build a good therapeutic alliance. They are therapists who do not hesitate to make linear statements while being systemic; they do not avoid giving prescriptions, even knowing that control is an illusion; they do not refuse to give advice, even knowing that advice does not change people. They are therapists who, to maintain clients at the centre of the therapeutic process, shares their own emotional experiences with clients; therapists who, before expressing their competence, make sure that clients feel comfortable and safe. This is a way of doing therapy that cannot be defined as eclectic, that is, without constraints, or artistic, as opposed to scientific, because, in the approach suggested here, creativity springs from the rigorous adoption of a method, the method of double description [Bateson 1979], which allows the therapists to always operate at 2 levels: that of their technical competency and that of the relationship with the client, which ultimately becomes the criterion based on which the therapists make their therapeutic choices.

Note

1 The extracts reported are taken from Fruggeri 2012, pp. 100–102.

References

Aronsson, K. and Cederborg, A.C. [1994], *Co-narration and voice in family therapy. Voicing, devoicing, and orchestration*, in Text, 1994, 14, pp. 345–370.

Aronsson, K. and Cekaite, A. [2011], *Activity contracts and directives in everyday family politics*, in Discourse & Society, 22, 2, pp. 1–18.

Bateson, G. [1972], *Steps to an ecology of mind*, New York, Chandler.

Bateson, G. [1979], *Mind and nature: a necessary unity*, New York, Bantam Books.

Byng-Hall, J. [1995], *Re-writing family scripts*, New York, Guilford Press.

Burnham, J. [2005], *Relational reflexivity: a tool for socially constructing therapeutic relationships*, in C. Flaskas, B. Mason and A. Perlesz (eds.), *The space between: experience, context, and process in the therapeutic relationships*, London, Karnac, pp. 1–18.

Burnham, J. [2012], *Developments in Social GRRRAAACCEEESSS: visible–invisible and voiced–unvoiced*, in B. Kruse (ed), *Culture and reflexivity in systemic psychotherapy*, Karnac, pp. 139–160.

Cingolani, S. [1995], *Come compromettere il bene alla ricerca del meglio. Appunti sulla patologia iatrogena ed i suoi rimedi da un punto di vista relazionale-sistemico*, in M. Bianciardi and U. Telfner (eds.), *Ammalarsi di Psicoterapia*, Milano, Franco Angeli, pp. 115–128.

Daniel, G. [2012], *With an exile's eye: developing positions of cultural reflexivity (with a bit of help from feminism)*, in B. Kruse (ed.), *Culture and reflexivity in systemic psychotherapy*, London, Karnac, pp. 91–113.

Ervin-Tripp, S.M., O'Connor, M.C. and Rosenberg, J. [1984], *Language and power in the family*, in M. Schulz and C. Kramerae (eds.), *Language and power*, Beverly Hills CA, Sage, pp. 117–135.

Friedlander, M.L., Escudero, V. and Heatherington, L. [2006], *Therapeutic alliances in couple and family therapy: an empirically informed guide to practice*, Washington DC, American Psychological Association.

Fruggeri, L. [1998], *Famiglie. Dinamiche interpersonali e processi psico-sociali*, Roma, Carocci.

Fruggeri, L. [2002], *Different levels of analysis in the supervisory process*, in D. Campbell and B. Mason (eds.), *Perspectives on supervision*, London, Karnac Books, pp. 3–20.

Fruggeri, L. [2012], *Different levels of psychotherapeutic competence*, in Journal of Family Therapy, 34, pp. 91–105.

Harré, R., Moghaddam, F.M., Pilkerton Cairnie, T., Rothbart, D. and Sabat, S.R. [2009], *Recent advances in positioning theory*, in Theory and Psychology, 19, pp. 5–31.

Helmeke, K.B. and Sprenkle, D.H. [2000], *Clients' perceptions of pivotal moments in couples therapy: a qualitative study of change in therapy*, in Journal of Marital and Family Therapy, 26, 4, pp. 469–483.

Hunsley, J., Aubry, T.D., Verstervelt, C.M. and Vito, D. [1999], *Comparing therapist and client perspectives on reasons for psychotherapy termination*, in Psychotherapy: Theory, Research, Practice, Training, 36, 4, pp. 380–388.

Jones, E. [2003], *Working with the "Self" of the therapist in consultation*, in Human Systems, n. 14, 1, pp. 7–16.

Lannamann, J. [1991], *Interpersonal communication. Research and ideological practice*, in Comunication Theory, 1991, 31, pp. 179–203.

Linell, P. [2009], *Rethinking language, mind and the world dialogically: interactional and contextual theories of human sense making*, Charlotte N.C, Information Age Publishing.

Ochs, E. and Taylor, C. [1996], *The "father knows best" dynamic in dinnertime narratives*, in K. Hall (ed.), *Gender articulated: language and the socially constructed Self*, London, Routledge, pp. 99–122.

Rober, P. [2005], *Family therapy as a dialogue of living persons*, in Journal of Marital and Family Therapy, 31, pp. 385–397.

Rober, P. [2011], *The therapists experiencing in family therapy*, in Journal of Marital and Family Therapy, 33, pp. 233–255.

Roy-Chowdhury, S. [2006], *How is the therapeutic relationship talked into being?*, in Journal of Family Therapy, 28, 2, pp. 153–174.

Shotter, J. [1987], *The social costruction of an "Us": problem of accountablity and narrtology*, in R. Burnett, P. McGhee and D. Clark (eds.), *Accounting for relationship and knowledge*, London, Mthuen, pp. 225–247.

Shotter, J. [2010], *Encountering the unique otherness of the other: exploring inner landscapes of feeling.* in Context, 111, pp. 25–30.

Shotter, J. [2015], *On being dialogical: an ethics of "attunement"*, in Context, 137, pp. 8–11.

Simon, G. [2016], *Systemic practice as systemic inquiry as transformative research*, in I. McCarthy and G. Simon, (eds.), *Systemic therapy as transformative practice*, Farnhill (UK), Everything is Connected Press, pp. 169–191.

Tannen, D. [2007], *You just don't understand. Women and men in conversation*, New York, Harper and Collins.

Tomm, K. [1987], *Interventive interviewing, part I: strategizing as a fourth guideline for the therapist*, in Family Process, 26, pp. 3–13.

Part III

Epistemological competency: the ability to change point of view

5 Reflexivity: becoming aware of one's own premises

Luigi Boscolo used to say to colleagues and trainees: "Don't fall in love with your hypotheses", and Gianfranco Cecchin echoed, "Don't be seduced by a model"[1].

Therapists' hypotheses about what maintains clients' problems and distress are methodological tools provisionally used to foster dialogue with clients. Systemic hypotheses are dynamic and involve the generation of a circular process triggered by clients' feedback and the subsequent adjustments made by the therapist (see Chapter 1). Nevertheless, as illustrated in Chapter 4, the application of techniques cannot be detached from the relational process that therapists and clients co-construct during the therapy sessions. In other words, the choice for one intervention rather than another is based on the analysis of the client–therapist interactions. This is a key characteristic of relational competency. In this sense, it should be emphasised that the very idea of changing the working hypothesis and of implementing it according to the analysis of the unfolding meaning-making process are implied in the concept of hypothesising itself. However, Boscolo's and Cecchin's warning is more radical; in fact, they don't invite therapists to merely change their hypothesis; they invite therapists to change their viewpoint or perspective whenever it is necessary. More specifically, Cecchin invited therapists to be "irreverent" towards their own ideas and opinions, and to be ready to change them if necessary [Cecchin, Lane and Ray 1992]. When should therapists change their viewpoints? They should do that in several situations, such as: when they cannot make sense of what is happening in the session; when they lose interest in the client's story and get bored; when they start feeling that the client is "resistant" or "too crazy to change"; or, on the other side, when they have the unpleasant feeling of being useless. These scenarios signal the therapist's impasse; these are the scenarios that describe therapists who have moved away from a relational/therapeutic position and are instead caught between two opposed sentiments: attribute responsibility for the lack of change either to the clients or to their own incompetence. It is the uncomfortable and barren position of blaming either the client or themselves.

In these situations, therapists need to practice the *epistemological competency*, namely the ability of therapists to change their own viewpoints. Every time

DOI: 10.4324/9781003278092-9

therapists feel they can't make any sense of what is going on in the life of clients or in their encounter with them, they need to change lenses or perspective to be able to see things in a different way, because what they see from the usual point of view may just maintain the problem as it is rather than introduce more novel ways of seeing and doing.

Why do we define the ability to change viewpoint as *epistemological* competency? We drew the term from Bateson.

> The interest that Bateson has for Epistemology with a capital E, that is, for "the science that studies the process of knowing" [Bateson and Bateson 1987, p. 20], leads him to deal with epistemologies with a lowercase e, that is, with local epistemologies, personal ones and those shared by specific social groups. This landing is not accidental, it is prefigured in the distinction he draws between epistemology understood as the philosophical study of "how knowledge is possible" and epistemology understood as the study of "how knowledge is done" [Bateson and Bateson 1987, p. 20]. And it is the option that he operates in favour of the second definition proposed, that is of an epistemology that is identified with the study of knowledge conceived as a process rather than as an object, which leads him to reflect on local epistemologies, on what he also called habits of thought, networks of presuppositions, preconceptions, premises and, in the first writings, apperceptive habits. These are all terms with which Bateson designates the organizing principles of knowledge that are reflexively connected to behaviours in the process of building reality.
>
> [Fruggeri 2021, p. 84]

In this sense, epistemological competency has to do with the awareness of one's own local epistemologies as a starting point for being able to take a different viewpoint.

Epistemological competency is very important for psychotherapists as it allows them to embrace multiple perspectives as a condition for collaborative, ethical, co-creative, and conscientious practices. Therapists implement the epistemological competency to protect their clients from the iatrogenic effects resulting from the rigidity of their models or interpretations. In this sense, epistemological competency does not pertain to the therapists' ability to change what they see or understand, but to change the lenses or perspective, namely, to change the *criteria* they use to make sense of the situation they are involved in. In this respect, Burnham and Harris [2002] draw the distinction between "making a hypothesis", which contains a specific idea, and "hypothesising", which entails the ability to construct, deconstruct, and reconstruct ideas.

However, deconstructing one's own ideas or observing phenomena from another viewpoint are not spontaneous operations, given the recursivity of observing systems [von Foerster 1981; Maturana and Varela 1980]. As Bateson specified:

In the natural history of the living human being, ontology and epistemology cannot be separated. His (commonly unconscious) beliefs about what sort of world it is will determine how he sees it and acts within it, and his ways of perceiving and acting will determine his beliefs about its nature. The living man is thus bound within a net of epistemological and ontological premises which – regardless of ultimate truth or falsity –become partially self-validating for him.

[Bateson 1972, p. 314]

Bateson's thoughts on epistemology have been sustained by experimental research on social cognition showing that when knowing, social actors tend to anchor what is not familiar to their previous knowledge [Jodelet 1984; Fiske and Taylor 1984].

Therefore, changing viewpoint means overcoming the rigidity that derives both from the conservatism of our cognitive functioning, and from the net of epistemological and ontological premises within which we are all bound. In this sense, epistemological competency is not given. Changing perspective and considering situations from a different point of view do not derive from the therapists' good will either. In fact, several factors prevent therapists from changing perspective or make it difficult: firstly, the is unawareness of one's own point of view or position, in other words, blindness to the categories that are used to observe and understand others' and one's own world; secondly, self-referentiality, that is, the belief that therapists know more than their clients; lastly, a simplistic and dualistic thinking that implies the existence of one truth. Nonetheless, antidotes to cognitive and interpretative rigidity are available to therapists. Unawareness can be contrasted through *self-reflexivity*, that is, reflecting upon the categories individuals use to know, observe, make sense of, and act in the world around them, which in Bateson's terms means reflecting upon "how knowledge is *done*" [Bateson and Bateson 1987, p. 20]. The loop of self-referentiality can be overcome by adopting a position of *curiosity*, namely becoming interested in the points of view of others [Cecchin 1987]. Lastly, simplistic and dualistic thinking can be overcome by practicing *complex thinking,* which implies acknowledging multiple points of view [Keeney 1983]. Self-reflexivity, curiosity, and complex thinking are the expressions of a competency that can be learned and practiced through specific epistemological exercises that can train therapists to understand how reality can be explained, described, and understood in several different ways. The three chapters included in this part of the book will address the three key components of the epistemological competency: this chapter is focused on self-reflexivity, Chapter 6 will illustrate complex thinking, and Chapter 7 will explore the notions of curiosity and decentring.

Exercising self-awareness

A central aspect in the definition of epistemological competency is becoming aware of one's own premises. As illustrated in Chapter 4, the therapist's knowledge is part of the interactive dynamic and can contribute to triggering positive and generative processes, but also negative and non-transformative ones. Therefore, self-reflexivity, i.e., reflecting upon one's own system of thinking, premises, and socio-cultural positions, is a key methodological principle that can assist therapists in evaluating the consequences of their knowledge at the social and interactional level.

In the 1970s and 1980s, some scholars warned psychotherapists against the use of diagnostic categories, language, and heuristic principles that could contribute to the social construction of psychopathology [Rosenhan 1973; Dell 1980; Boscolo and Cecchin 1983; Watzlawick 1984; Anderson, Goolishian and Winderman 1986]. Afterwards, the debate mainly focused on the psychotherapists' language. For instance, in conversations with colleagues or in writing, the term "patient" has been associated with the term "designated" to stress that the member who has been identified as "problematic" signals, instead, that the problem concerns the whole family. Gradually the term "patient" has been abandoned, and it has been replaced with the term "client", to acknowledge the subjectivity of the person seeking help. Also, the terms "therapy", "cure", and "problem", which evoked a bio-medical, lineal approach, have been replaced with terms such as "conversation", "narration", and "concern", to consistently refer to an approach based on circularity, social relations, and communication processes. In general, traditional diagnostic categories have been questioned for their risk of labelling clients and objectifying their difficulties [Boscolo *et al.* 1987].

However, self-reflection should not be confined to the use of technical or scientific language only. In fact, therapists belong to both professional and sociocultural communities, and as such, their practice is not only guided by scientific knowledge but also by "common sense" knowledge, which they often are unaware of. According to Gramsci [1992], common sense is characterized by a total and unlimited adherence to a world view that is expressed through a blind and irrational obedience to indemonstrable and non-scientific principles and precepts. Common sense is never questioned; it is considered an absolute truth. In fact, it is the expression of the dominant class. Therapists, like any other social actor, share social representations, prejudices, stereotypes, implicit theories, and beliefs with the communities they belong to. In this sense, they also share a form of knowledge that is taken for granted. Common sense knowledge corresponds to dominant discourses, supports the social system, and is sustained by it. As Bateson underlined:

> The ideas [that people share] about nature, however fantastic, are supported by their social system; conversely, the social system is supported by their ideas of nature. It thus becomes very difficult for the people, so doubly guided, to change their view either of nature or of the social system. For the benefits of stability, they pay the price of rigidity, living, as all human beings must, in an enormously complex network of mutually supporting presuppositions.
>
> [Bateson 1979, p. 154]

This type of shared thinking is unknowingly used to understand who we are, who others are, and the world around us, without questioning the status quo. In common sense knowledge, diversity, originality, and uniqueness are not acknowledged; they are rather considered deviations or distortions to be corrected. Common sense has only one truth, so it makes people blind to other ways of understanding "reality". Nevertheless, therapists may use common sense knowledge in their practice without being aware of it. Self-reflexivity allows therapists to critically analyse their implicit theories, socio-cultural premises, and representations. In this sense, it is a key methodological principle for the development of epistemological competency that helps therapists to overcome interpretative rigidity. The case example reported below shows how self-reflexivity allows therapists to interrupt the loops that make them feel stuck and foster the therapeutic process with new ideas.

Lulia contacts a therapist privately for her teenage daughter Alida, who is 16 years old. Lulia told the therapist that over the last 2 years Alida has been reluctant to interact with people to the extent that she refused to go to school and eventually missed 2 years of school. Initially the mother thought that Alida did not study because she was just lazy; thus, she punished her for not going to school. However, that did not solve the problem. Then, Lulia decided to contact the psychologists working in the healthcare service, who diagnosed Alida with a social phobia. Only at that moment did the mother understand that her daughter had a psychological problem, and she informed Alida's teachers about it. Since then, Alida has gone to school and has worked hard to improve her school attainment. At the time of the first interview with the therapist, Alida attended the first year of a secondary school. She was doing well and had a group of friends. The teenager acknowledged that things had improved, but she felt she needed psychological support and asked her mother to see a psychologist.

In the first interview conducted with both Alida and her mother, Alida listened to her mother, rarely spoke, and answered the therapist's questions with a faint voice. Also, given that she had always been considered as listless and negligent in school, she appeared sensitive to judgements and somewhat defensive. Nonetheless, she reaffirmed the willingness to start individual therapy. In the subsequent sessions, the therapist focused on the creation of a secure relational context and of an emotional connection with Alida (see Chapter 3) to allow her to feel comfortable and talk about her problems without feeling judged.

The teenager told the therapist that her father died for a heart attack 5 years earlier. Since then, things had changed radically in her family. Her parents used to have many friends thanks to the contacts that her father used to maintain; after his death, friends disappeared. Alida and her mother felt lonely and became very close in supporting each other. The two of them never talked about the loss of her father. The therapist formulated the hypotheses that Alida's social phobia kept the mother busy: Lulia devoted herself to caring for Alida, thereby limiting both her daughter's and her own autonomy. Building upon this hypothesis, the therapist worked to help Alida to explore the loss of her father and talk to her mother about this in order to allow them to continue with their individual life projects.

After almost 1 year of therapy, the situation between Alida and Lulia had greatly improved: Alida continued to go out with her friends and was able to successfully finish the second year of secondary school. The relationship between Alida and the therapist was good. After the school summer break, Alida told the therapist she had decided not to go back to school[2]; however, she was concerned about this choice since she feared she could be negatively judged and could be pushed to do something she did not want to do. The therapist knew that the school was still a difficult environment for Alida, since it limited the teenager's potential and made her feel deeply inadequate. Therefore, the therapist decided to support Alida in communicating her choice to her mother.

However, in subsequent sessions the therapist began to feel concerned for Alida as well as helpless herself: after leaving school, Alida was not looking for jobs. Instead, she was volunteering for a charity involved with people with disabilities. The therapist believed that finding a job was an essential condition for Alida's autonomy; therefore, she centred the interviews on that topic. However, whenever the therapist brought up the job issue, Alida became silent and looked like the inadequate teenager of the early sessions.

The therapist was concerned about this case; therefore, she decided to ask for peer supervision. What did the therapist not see? What was the premise that made her blind? During the reflection with colleagues, the therapist realised that she was basing her intervention on the rigid premise that autonomy can be reached only through a job. The therapist's premise is shared in the professional world: having a job is considered a fundamental achievement in individuals' psychosocial development [Kaneklin and Gozzoli 2011]. However, curious therapists should be ready to challenge their professional ideas and ask themselves how useful they are to the client [Hedges 2005, p. 73]. The premise that autonomy could be achieved only through a job prevented the therapist from seeing that Alida was developing her autonomy through her commitment to volunteering. In fact, while volunteering, the teenager was creating social relationships, was carrying out tasks and duties, and was taking responsibility. The therapist embraced this new perspective and met with Alida. During the session, the therapist apologised with Alida for having been focused on the job issue and not seeing how volunteering had been an important training experience for her. Also, she appreciated Alida's ability to find that option as a way to become independent. Alida was very attentive, appeared reassured by the therapist's words, and appreciated the fact that the therapist acknowledged her competence. The subsequent sessions went very well. Alida decided to apply for government funding for youth wanting to work for charities, and after a couple of months, both Alida and the therapist agreed it was time to conclude the therapy.

Gianfranco Cecchin argued that a certain dose of irreverence [Cecchin, Lane and Ray 1992] is necessary to be able to reflect upon oneself. In other words, therapists should become aware of the temporary nature of their viewpoints, since meanings change according to the context and the moment in which those viewpoints have been generated: self-reflexivity builds upon this awareness. Therefore, the starting point for the development of a self-reflexive position is acknowledging that every phenomenon can be observed from multiple points of view; this implies challenging one's own premises. Going back to the case example illustrated above, during the peer supervision session, the therapist went through a reflexive process that: (1) started with consideration of the ideas that guided the creation of the relationship with her client, (2) continued with the acknowledgement that those ideas were not the truth, but only one possible point of view among others, and (3) concluded with the exploration of other possible points of view. This self-reflexive process experienced during supervision can be considered a model for personal reflection to exercise whenever therapists feel they are going into a situation of impasse. However, as an individual practice, self-reflexivity might prove ineffective if it drifts back to self-reference. Self-reflexivity can be more effectively practiced and learned in conversations with other people, when listening to others' self-reflections, in dialogue with colleagues, and in all situations in which therapists are confronted with multiple points of view. Lastly, self-reflexivity can be exercised by analysing therapists' actions, in particular by observing what they do [Balestra and Fruggeri 2016]. Roy-Chowdhury [2003] pointed out that meticulous analysis of therapy session transcripts highlighted the implicit theories embedded in therapists' actions, thereby making them aware of their points of view. However, sometimes cognitive awareness is not enough to trigger a self-reflexive process: sometimes it is only through reflection on the therapists' emotions, that is, on what they "feel", that it is possible for therapists to understand their position in the therapeutic process [Krause 1993; Lini and Bertrando 2020].

Emotions and self-reflexivity

Therapists' emotions can become overwhelming to the extent that they become responsible for creating a situation of impasse. In these cases, reflexivity is more easily implemented through analogic languages since emotions might block thoughts. This is what happened in the case illustrated below.

In a supervision session, Sophia, one of the trainees of a master course in systemic psychotherapy, described a clinical case she found particularly difficult to deal with. The case concerned individual therapy she provided for a client, Paola, during the clinical hours of the training. Paola was a young woman who had trouble keeping stable romantic relationships, since she did not feel accepted by the men she dated. She reported feeling belittled and like a failure, especially when she compared herself with her married sister. Paola told the therapist she was born by accident and her parents married because her mother was pregnant with her. Before getting married, her father wanted to make sure Paola was his biological daughter. Her grandmother on her mother's side had her daughter (Paola's mother) with a married man, who never acknowledged her as his child; this was never spoken about in her family despite everybody knowing it. The grandmother, the mother, and Paola were very close. Paola had a conflictual relationship with her father, who put Paola in charge of her mother, who had physical problems. The mother was ambivalent towards Paola: on the one hand, she acknowledged Paola's need for autonomy; on the other hand, she continually asked for support with travelling and attending medical visits.

During the supervisory session, Sophia reported that when she had invited Paola to ask her father and sister to become more responsible for her mother's care, she started to cry and said she could not abandon her mother. Paola showed intense anger and frustration. Sophia presented this case since she believed she was unable to create a good relationship with Paola. According to Sophia, Paola was very confused and sad; in the few sessions they had together, they were unable to create a good therapeutic alliance since Paola seemed afraid of being judged. The group of trainees thought that, like Paola, Sophia looked confused and sad: when her colleagues gave her feedback, she defended her point of view and interventions as if she felt judged by her colleagues, as well as belittled and frustrated. However, the trainees also felt they were unable to help Sophia to overcome this impasse.

This is the moment when a different language is needed to help Sophia to distance herself from the emotional reactions of anger and frustration derived from the impact of Paola's case on her. The trainer asks Sophia's colleagues to role-play Paola's family members: Paola, the mother, the father, the sister and her husband, and the grandparents from Paola's mother's and father's side. Sophia is invited to place the colleagues acting as family members in different parts of the room, choosing their distance, their postures, and the direction of their gazes. In so doing, Sophia can represent her idea of Paola's family and of the relationships among her client's family members. She puts the maternal grandmother, the mother, and Paola very close, as if in a circle. The maternal grandfather and Paola's father are positioned with their backs to both of their wives and Paola. Paola's sister, her husband, and the paternal grandparents are distant from the others. Once Sophia is done with positioning the family members, she is invited to observe and to listen to what she is feeling without sharing it with the group. Then, the trainer asks each "actor" to share how they feel in the position assigned by Sophia. Based on their answers, the actors are invited to move in the room to take a position that can make them feel better. The actors move around the room until they find a more comfortable position. Thus, the representation of Paola's family starts to change. Sophia, in her role of observer, looks at the creation of a new family configuration and listens to her emotions and to the emotions shared by the actors.

The new configuration starts with the movement of the father, who says he does not feel comfortable in that position as he cannot see his family: neither his wife nor his daughters. Thus, he gets closer to his wife, and from that position he can also see his daughters. The person playing the sister says she feels too far from the rest of the family; thus, she moves closer to Paola, who, in turn, says she feels trapped between her mother and grandmother. She is happy that her father is now closer, as well as her sister; therefore, she decides to move next to her. The trainee playing the mother says she is happy to have her husband next to her and her daughters in front of her, but she is concerned for her mother, who is alone. At this point, the maternal grandfather moves next to Paola's grandmother. The trainer asks the actors how they feel; they all answer that they feel better in the new configuration.

"Visualizing" relationships can be more effective than just listening to the "description" of relationships since it is possible to see what the cognitive channel does not allow one to see. In fact, Sophia begins to see and listen to something she was unable to either see or listen to earlier; namely that the narration can change and that everybody can contribute to narrate a new story in their own time. Sophia realizes that she confused the "map with the territory": in other words, she thought that Paola's "loyalty" to her mother was an inevitable destiny, which spanned three generations since Paola's mother was also bound to the loyalty to her mother, as if the three women had to hold together to protect themselves from the shame of the "illegitimate" births. Loyalty is a positive feeling; however, it becomes dysfunctional if it acquires rigid connotations, and it traps both the client and the therapist within a prefigured path from which there is no escape. With this new vision, Sophia decides to reflect with Paola on the sense of guilt, which might emerge from breaching the family loyalty. In other words, thanks to the colleagues' role-play, Sophia was able to refocus the goals of the therapy and create a new narrative that could highlight the resources present in the family system.

Sometimes, the feeling of being "emotionally stuck" connects with experiences concerning the therapists' deutero-learnings, that is, legacy of cultural, social, political, and familial themes, meanings and patterns of interaction that inform their psychological and relational being. These experiences can resurface in the relationship with clients and unwittingly lead to blind spots. In this sense, self-reflexivity can be learned by using specific techniques and by undergoing a process of self-awareness that trains therapists to acknowledge the emotions emerging in the therapeutic contexts and identify those that can lead to an impasse (see Box 5.1).

Box 5.1   The therapist's self between emotions and self-reflexivity by Anna Castellucci

The training program for psychotherapists carried out at the Bologna Centre for Family Therapy (CBTF) in Bologna (Italy) includes a program aimed at developing a self-reflexive competency on parts of the self that are often not acknowledged or even denied, which however can hinder the construction of generative relationships with clients. The program employs a methodology based on the integration of different techniques: the main tool of the systemic therapist, that of asking questions, is flanked by techniques such as psycho-genealogy, dialogue of voices, dramatization, and autobiographical writing.

Through the exercise of the "heraldic shield", during the first year we focus on the beliefs that everyone learns growing up in their family of origin. The exercise involves identifying a motto that defines in an analogical way the specificity of the family and its member's way of life. Mottos like "Stay one step behind", "Whoever stops is lost", "Make yourself worthy", and "Take the maximum from everything", just to name a few, talk about us, about how we move in the world. Monitoring the trainees' progress involves observing if and how the motto changes during training. Movements such as: from "Stay one step back" to "Open yourself to new ideas", from "Always aim high" to "Things come to those who can wait", from "There is always hope" to "Change is an act of courage" show that students are on a journey for new explorations around their own Self.

The reflection on one's motto is deepened during the second year of training with the work on the genogram. The work proposed at the CBTF contemplates an integration of the classical method of genogram [Carter and McGoldrick 1988] with the ideas of psychogenealogy introduced by Schutzenberger [2014]. In line with this integration, the construction of the genogram unravels starting from a question that the subject feels is relevant today to reflect and comment on the family tree, starting from a relevant theme in current life. From this perspective it is not so important to identify and isolate the "real" content of the transgenerational experience of the family (myths, rules, rituals, and secrets), but the meaning it assumes in the relationship between the family myth and the individual myth. "The lesson of systemics and psychogenealogy" explains Miszczyszyn, "is to teach the person to pay off the debt by aligning herself not with the sense of guilt or with the logic of the preservation of suffering but respecting the existential needs of evolution and affirmation of the vital energy" [2008, p. 45].

The journey continues in the third year with a module entitled "Me, my family, and the invisible alliances". In particular, the issues high-lighted in the exploration of the family tree are resumed to address them from a different perspective and to monitor if, over the course of a year, they have changed. In this case we explore the emotions connected to difficulties encountered in some areas of life, analysing if there are connections with episodes that occurred to an ancestor present in our family tree. To do this, masks made by an Argentine craftsman are used. On the one hand, masks conceal and on the other reveal and can be, in this sense, an excellent metaphor to stimulate self-observation and introspection. The exercise aims to stimulate a different perception of oneself through what one imagines that others see in us through the mask. It is the gaze of the Other on us that allows us to identify and recognize ourselves. The mask somehow makes us feel protected and at the same time stripped; in any case, it represents an opportunity to observe ourselves through whoever looks at us.

The module "Knowing and integrating one's Selves", scheduled for the fourth year, introduces questions and reflections on which parts of us (Self) we have most developed and how these have become repetitive patterns. The aim is to become aware of the many different "Selves" that alternate in guiding our daily life to make them become a resource in therapeutic work.

The different exercises include an exploration of culture and of the socio-political context in which the events narrated have occurred.

Self-reflexivity and social positioning

As we have discussed in the previous paragraphs, thanks to self-reflexivity, therapists can become aware of the beliefs, prejudices, stereotypes, biases, assumptions, and emotions that might interfere with their creativity and ability to join dialogically the clients' subjectivity. But both clients and therapists are rooted in socio-cultural contexts, and as such, they are also the embodiments of social differences. The importance of being aware of, sensitive to, and competent in working with issues of social differences that entail power relationships between therapists and clients has been stressed lately by many authors (see the following). From this perspective, therapists' self-reflexivity implies to reflect upon their own and their clients' embodied positions with respect to these issues. In this case, the questions that foster therapists' self-reflexivity are the following ones: How do social differences between therapists and clients or trainers and trainees affect the therapeutic/learning relationship? How do therapists perceive the differences that they embody? How do they deal with such differences and with the power relation that they may entail? What feedback do therapists receive about themselves from their clients with respect to how they are positioned in the social context?

Daniel [2012] invites therapists to reflect on the feedback they receive about themselves as cultural/gendered beings. "Viewing ourselves with the eyes of others" is a good exercise that provides therapists with the possibility to learn about their positions in the power relationships generated by cultural differences and, thus, to incorporate them in the process of change involving both therapists and clients.

Burnham, Alvis Palma and Whitehouse [2008] have argued how training courses should help trainees to develop the ability to explore social issues such as gender, geography, religion, age, ability, class, culture, ethnicity, employment, education, sexuality, sexual orientation, and spirituality (GGRAACC-EEESS), and how to use them in their relationship with clients. According to these authors, all issues of social differences are continuously relevant and influential in the co-creation of contexts for therapy and learning. They are always present; yet, not all issues are visible and voiced. They point out how some social differences are visible and voiced, whereas others may be visible and unvoiced; or invisible and voiced as well as invisible and unvoiced, and all movements in between [see also Burnham, 2012]. Because of this variability, therapists may not become aware of the social differences that contribute to create relationships in therapeutic and learning contexts. So, the authors propose a set of questions that foster self-reflection on social issues to help therapists deal with them.

- What similarities/differences are visible/voiced?
- What similarities/differences are visible/unvoiced?
- What similarities/differences am I aware of in this moment/relationship?
- What differences do we want to name and what differences do we want to silence?
- What differences do we want to preserve and what differences do we want to integrate?
- What is the need in the moment, and does this require emphasizing difference or integration? [Burnham *et al.* 2008, pp. 538–539].

These questions suggest that self-reflexivity is an activity that must be contextualized; in fact, "voicing the unvoiced, or bringing the invisible into the conversation might contribute to transparency that is therapeutic, or exposure that becomes unhelpful" [Burnham 2012, p. 147].

In this respect, the discussion about self-disclosure of therapists who identify as transgender is very interesting and full of inspiring ideas. Disclosure of a therapist's transgender identity has not yet been systematically studied, and since results are contradictory (some authors see it as detrimental to the therapeutic alliance, whereas others note that it can strengthen the therapist–client relationship), most authors underline how decisions about self-disclosure must be examined within the context in which the therapist operates. In this sense, some contributions are particularly interesting for how they describe the complexity of the decision-making process about self-disclosure. Within such a complexity, context and self-reflexivity are the key words: context because it is only by analysing the contingent relational context that therapists can evaluate whether the disclosure can be helpful or not, and self-reflectivity is central in monitoring the impact of self-disclosure on the ongoing therapeutic process [Blumer and Barbachano 2008; Shipman and Martin 2017].

The issue of therapists' self-disclosure is, in general, central in contemporary systemic therapy. A psychotherapeutic encounter is characterized by the intersection of different identities held by therapists and clients, and these identities are meaningful with respect to the development of the therapeutic process, especially those associated with privilege and power. For this reason, it might be helpful for therapists to initiate a conversation with clients about similarities and differences in race, ethnicity, gender, class, sexual orientation, and religion, and to reflect on how they may influence the therapeutic process. In this respect, Dee Watts-Jones [2010] proposes a very interesting reflection about the circumstances when a dialogue on the identities held by therapists and clients may be beneficial. Three assumptions are at the base of her work. First, therapists should feel comfortable to address any issue in order to create a context in which clients feel safe to explore it. The second assumption is that identities of therapists and clients should be a topic of conversation since they are like a lens through which therapists and clients understand the world, and as such, they matter in the therapy process, particularly identities associated with social advantage/disadvantage and power. Finally, Dee Watts-Jones underlines how oppression is infused into systems of thought, associations, and values, implicit and explicit, and institutional and cultural practices; thus, issues of oppression are always relevant in therapy. Training and supervision can nurture through self-reflexivity the ability to deal in a comfortable way with the issues connected to intersectionality present in therapy encounters and processes.

Self-reflexivity on social differences also entails therapists being aware of the language they use. Prejudices, stereotypes, and inequality are constructed and maintained through language, daily verbal and non-verbal language. Race, gender, and sexuality related discourses can be constructed by participants in family and couple therapy without any awareness. This would make the power issues connected to social differences invisible, thus unavailable to address in the therapeutic conversation. By talking of social differences-related discourses, we refer to the definition proposed by Janusz and colleagues [Janusz, Jozefik and Perakila 2018, p. 437], that is, "all social practices – verbal or embodied – that in a given moment can evoke and make relevant assumptions about women and men", but also about GBLT+ community members or about peoples belonging to different ethnic groups or any other social group, and to all the possible intersections among them. From this point of view, self-reflexivity implies making visible the assumptions about social differences embedded in therapeutic discourses.

In particular, an invitation to self-reflexivity comes from systemic psychotherapists involved in the development of decolonising systemic practices (See issue 44,1 of the *Journal of Family Therapy*). Racism is structural in our society: public policies, institutional practices, social and cultural representations, norms and dominant values, and language perpetuate racial group inequality, associating privileges with "whiteness" and disadvantages with "colours" and especially with "blackness". In order to develop a critical consciousness in relation to structural racism, psychotherapists need to start with themselves. As proposed by Chin, Hughes and Miller [2022], therapists can make a decolonizing shift in their practice, if they explore the impact of racism on themselves, their life, and their relationships, and reflect on how they position themselves in a context of structural racism and on how they respond to it.

Moreover, given the pervasiveness of heterosexism, straight therapists who work with LGBT+ individuals, couples, or families should systematically assess homophobic and heterosexist assumptions embedded in both personal attitudes, professional theory, language, and practice [Bernstein 2000]. Straight therapists who fail to invest in personal exploration before working with LGBT+ clients are at risk for potentially harming them because they may unknowingly contribute to recreating a heteronormative environment in the therapeutic context [Shelton and Delgado-Romero 2011]. To avoid this, they are invited to develop a knowledge of the main issues concerning such a community and, more important, to reflect upon their own values, biases, and prejudices about sex, gender, and sexual orientation, and on how these biases can affect interactions with clients [Godfrey *et al.* 2006]. Self-reflexivity is the condition for straight therapists to create a therapeutic context within which they can help to correct the internalized homophobia and heterosexism eventually experienced by clients, but also to take a further step of advocacy and contribute to undo societal institutional heteronormativity [Cooper 2015].

We will discuss these issues further in Chapter 10.

Notes

1 Luigi Boscolo and Gianfranco Cecchin are Italian therapists known worldwide for having pioneered the application of the systemic approach to psychotherapy. Throughout the 1980s and the 1990s, they trained hundreds of therapists in different countries. Their clinical skills, together with the innovations of their approach, have influenced clinical practitioners all over the world. Cecchin died in a car accident in 2004, while Boscolo passed away after an illness in 2015.
2 The reader should be aware that in Italy school obligation ends at the accomplishment of 10th grade, after which a youngster can decide to stop school and find a job. So, Alida's decision must not be considered a drop out from school, but the choice of an option provided by the system.

References

Anderson, H., Goolishian, H. and Winderman, L. [1986], *Problem determined systems: toward a transformation in family therapy*, in Journal of Strategic and Systemic Therapies, 5, pp. 14–19.

Balestra, F. and Fruggeri, L. [2016], *Paths to transformative conversations*, in G. Simon and I. McCarthy (eds.), *Systemic therapy as transformative practice*, Farnhill UK, Everything Is Connected Press, pp. 316–330.

Bateson, G. [1972], *Steps to an ecology of mind*, New York, Chandler.

Bateson, G. [1979], *Mind and nature: a necessary unity*, New York, Bantam Books.

Bateson, G. and Bateson, M.C. [1987], *Angels fear*, New York, Macmillan;

Bernstein, A. [2000] *Straight therapists working with lesbians and gays in family therapy*, in Journal of Marital and Family Therapy, 26, 4, pp. 443–454

Blumer, M.L.C. and Barbachano, J.M. [2008], *Valuing the gender-variant therapist: therapeutic experiences, tools, and implications of a female-to-male trans-variant clinician*, in Journal of Feminist Family Therapy, 20, 1, pp.46–65.

Boscolo, L. and Cecchin, G. [1983], *La psicoterapia e le sue finalità*, in M. Malagoli Togliatti and U. Telfener (eds.), *La terapia sistemica*, Roma, Astrolabio, pp. 89–97.

Boscolo, L., Cecchin, G., Hoffman, L. and Penn, P. [1987], *Milan systemic family therapy*, New York, Basic Books.

Burnham, J. and Harris, Q. [2002] *Cultural issues in supervision*, in D. Campbell and B. Mason (eds.), *Perspectives in supervision*, London, Karnak, pp. 21–41.

Burnham, J., Alvis Palma, D. and Whitehouse, L. [2008], *Learning as a context for differences, and differences as a context for learning*, in Journal of Family Therapy, 30, 4, pp. 529–542.

Burnham, J., and Kruse, B. [2012], *Developments in social GRRRAAACCEEESSS: visible-invisible and voiced-unvoiced*, in B. Kruse (ed.), *Culture and reflexivity in systemic psychotherapy*, London, Karnac, pp. 139–160.

Carter, B. and McGoldrick, M. (eds.) [1988], *The changing family life cycle: a framework for family therapy* (2nd ed.), New York, Gardner Press.

Cecchin, G. [1987], *Hypothesizing, circularity, and neutrality revisited: an invitation to curiosity*, in Family Process, 26, 4, pp. 405–413.

Cecchin, G., Lane, G. and Ray, W.A. [1992], *Irreverence: a strategy for therapists' survival*, London, Karnac Books.

Chin, J., Hughes, G. and Miller, A. [2022] *Examining our own relationships to racism as the foundation of decolonising systemic practices. "No time like the present"*, in Journal of Family Therapy, 44, 1, pp. 76–90.

Cooper, M.A. [2015], *Sexual orientation competence: psychologists' perceived competence and relationships to multicultural competence, training, engagement, and exposure to lesbian, gay, and bisexual individuals*, Seton Hall University, Dissertations and Theses (ETDs).

Daniel, G. [2012], *With an exile's eye: developing positions of cultural reflexivity (with a bit of help from feminism)*, in B. Kruse (ed.), *Culture and reflexivity in systemic psychotherapy*, London, Karnac Books, pp. 91–113.

Dee Watts-Jones, T. [2010], *Location of self: opening the door to dialogue on intersectionality in the therapy process*, in Family Process, 49, 3, pp. 405–420.

Dell, P. [1980], *Researching the family theories of schizophrenia: an exercise in epistemological confusion*, in Family Process, 19, pp. 321–335.

Fiske, S.T. and Taylor, S.E. [1984], *Social cognition*, Usa-Canada, Addison-Wesley Publishing Company.

Fruggeri, L. [2021] *Social research as a process of interaction*, in Murmurations: Journal of Transformative Practice, 3, 2, pp. 81–99 10.28963/3.2.6

Gramsci, A. [1992], *Prison notebooks*, NY, Columbia University Press.

Godfrey, K., Haddock, S.A., Fisher, A. and Lund, L. [2006], *Essential components of curricula for preparing therapists to work effectively with lesbian, gay, and bisexual clients: a Delphi study*, in Journal of Marital and Family Therapy, 32, 4, pp. 491–504.

Hedges, F. [2005], *An introduction to systemic therapy with individuals. A social constructionist approach*, London, Palgrave Macmillan.

Janusz, B., Jozefik B. and Perakila A. [2018], *Gender-related issues in couple therapists' internal voices and interactional practices*, in Australian and New Zealand Journal of Family Therapy, 39, pp. 436–449.

Jodelet, D. [1984], *Représentations sociales: phénomène, concepts et théorie*, in S. Moscovici (ed.) *Psychologie sociale*, Paris, Press Universitaire de France.

Kaneklin, C. and Gozzoli, C. [2011], *Identità adulta al lavoro e cultura della flessibilità*, in C. Regaglia and E. Marta (eds.), *Identità in relazione. Le sfide odierne dell'essere adulto*, Milano, McGrow-Hill, pp. 53–71.

Keeney, B.P. [1983], *Aesthetics of change*, New York, Guilford Press.

Krause, I.B. [1993] *Anthropology and family therapy: a case for emotions*, in Journal of Family Therapy, 15, pp. 35–56.

Lini, C. and Bertrando, P. [2020], *Finding one's place: emotions and positioning in systemic-dialogical therapy*, in Journal of Family Therapy, 42, 2, pp. 204–221.

Maturana, H. and Varela, F. [1980], *Autopoiesis and cognition*, Dordrecht Holland, Reide.

Miszczyszyn, A. [2008], *Il potere delle radici*, Milano, Urra Edizioni.

Rosenhan, D. [1973], *On being sane in insane places*, in Science, 179, pp. 250–258.

Roy-Chowdhury, S. [2003], *Knowing the unknowable: what constitutes evidence in family therapy?*, in Journal of Family Therapy, 25, pp. 64–85.

Schutzenberger, A.A. [2014], *The ancestor syndrome: transgenerational psychotherapy and the hidden links in the family tree*. London, Routledge.

Shelton, K. and Delgado-Romero, E.A. [2011], *Sexual orientation microaggressions: the experience of lesbian, gay, bisexual, and queer clients in psychotherapy*, in Journal of Counseling Psychology, 58, 2, pp. 210–221.

Shipman D. and Martin T. [2017], *Clinical and supervisory considerations for transgender therapists: implications for working with clients*, in Journal of Marital and Family Therapy, 45, 1, pp. 92–105.

von Foerster, H. [1981], *Observing systems*, Seaside CA, Intersystems Publications.

Watzlawick, P. (ed) [1984], *The invented reality*, New York, Norton.

6 Complex thinking: the exploration of different perspectives

Self-reflexivity, discussed in the previous chapter, is only one dimension of epistemological competency, that is the ability to change point of view. In order "to see things in a different way", as the notion of epistemological competency suggests doing, therapists need to have access to "different ways of looking". Yet, the exploration of different perspectives doesn't come naturally in western cultures which are oriented to the search for "one truth". Therapists of the western world need to develop such an attitude through a specific training that can educate them to implement complex thinking.

This chapter will describe specific epistemological exercises on how "reality" can be explained, described, understood in different ways, namely: 1) Connecting the opposites, that is taking a "both ... and" instead of an "either ... or ... " perspective; 2) Deconstructing the dominant ideas that are usually taken for granted and, as such, might reveal to be oppressive; 3) Providing multiple descriptions of the same phenomenon; 4) Practicing divergent thinking which celebrates novelties and resources instead of traditions and deficiencies.

Practicing complementarity: connecting the opposites

Bateson [1979, p. 208] applied "the term complementarity to interactional sequences in which the actions of A and B were different but mutually fitted each other (e.g., dominance/submission, dependence/nurturance, exhibitionism/spectatorship)". The main characteristic of these pairs is that one element cannot exist without the other; they influence and depend on one another, such as: stability/change, individual/relationship, and many others [see, Keeney 1983, p. 93]. However, people adopting a dualistic epistemology, which is typical of western cultures, would see these pairs as composed of opposite elements defined by the logic of *either ... or*: if Mary is autonomous, she cannot be dependent; if a system changes, it cannot remain the same; if Tom is strong, he cannot be weak; a selfish person cannot be altruistic[1] and so on.

Following Bateson's invitation to look for the "pattern which connects", apparently opposite pairs can be correlated, or in Varela's terms [1979] "embricated", which means that one pole emerges from the relationship with the other, in such a way that A cannot exist without B. Consider the

DOI: 10.4324/9781003278092-10

pair stability/change: a system can change only starting from a situation of stability; similarly, the stability of a system is maintained through the transformations made to respond to internal and external solicitations to change. For instance, families can be the same (i.e., maintain their identity throughout the years) because of the capacity of the system to adjust to the changes of their members and the transformations of the social and cultural contexts in which they live. The interconnection between autonomy and dependence has been elegantly explained by Attachment Theory, showing that the development of an individual's autonomy is possible when a secure relational context (based on children's dependence from their carers) is provided. The pair individual/relationship is another example of complementary elements, as shown by research on identity development: a relationship is a liaison between two individuals, whose individuality is constructed through the interaction with others in social contexts [Luyckx and Vignoles 2012]. Research studies have shown that altruism originates also from selfish motivations since being proactive and caring for others has a positive impact on the Self [Batson *et al.* 1981]. Similarly, being "selfish" in terms of caring for oneself and aiming for self-realization can allow others to become independent and follow their aspirations. Family therapists are very familiar with the opposite dynamic: one member of the family is entirely dedicated to other members binding them in a relationship that doesn't leave space for anybody's autonomy and individuation. Individual and group dimensions are interconnected aspects of family functioning: promoting individuals' autonomy cannot be pursued at the expense of cohesion among family members; otherwise, there would be no family. Similarly, caring for mutual relationships and the sense of belonging to a group (or a family) cannot prevent members of a family from persuing their autonomy and independence [Fruggeri 1998]. Strength and weakness are two faces of the same coin: strong persons know how to express their weaknesses and to ask for help, whereas persons who are not allowed to show their weaknesses can be very vulnerable because they cannot count on the help for which they are not able to ask [Brown 2015]. Being a strong or a weak person are roles often rigidly played out by family members. Therapists can help family members to see the complementarity of strength/weakness, thereby allowing them to see each other in a different light. Even conflict and bonding, seemingly opposite pairs, can be considered as interdependent: therapists working with highly conflictual divorced couples are quite familiar with this situation since through conflict partners continue to be bonded in a toxic but inextricable way. Taken together, these examples show that the "opposite pairs" cannot be separated; rather, they can be considered as different punctuations of the same complex phenomenon. Practicing to "see" both punctuations allows therapists to develop an approach that fosters the analysis of phenomena from multiple points of view. Such an approach contributes to the development of epistemological competency, namely the ability to "to see things in a different way" and to overcome rigid interpretations that can lead to therapeutic impasse. Consider the case illustrated below.

Margaret and James are respectively 48 and 50 years old; they have been married for 20 years and have two children aged 18 and 17 years. James contacts a therapist since over the last year the relationship with his wife has become critical. He told the therapist that Margaret believes he is cheating on her with a younger woman he met at a sports club. Margaret and James used to be professional swimmers and still attend the sports club where they met 25 years ago. James is a swimming instructor, and Margaret oversees the club administration. Almost 1 year and a half ago, a 20-year-old woman named Glenn started the swimming course that James was instructing. Margaret says she did not notice anything suspicious at the beginning, but after some months she noticed some changes in the way James approached her: he was more distant and silent and was always speaking on the phone. Also, she noticed that James and Glenn often talked standing by the swimming pool; furthermore, some colleagues made jokes about James and Glenn flirting. While listening to Margaret's story, James looks astonished and denies everything his wife says. He claims he would never have done anything like that, especially with such a young woman of almost the same age as their daughter. He stresses he cannot stand his wife's accusations anymore. In fact, because of her obsession with Glenn, she is making their lives miserable. He does not know what to do to prove that what Margaret thinks is not true. For this reason, they have decided to seek help from a therapist. They add that their children are often present when they fight; the couple tends to avoid doing that in front of them, but it is difficult given the high frequency of their arguments.

The partners say they used to get along very well; however, there has been another critical moment for the couple. When their children were little, Margaret felt very lonely: James was very busy with swimming competitions while she quit her job to look after the children. Nonetheless, at that time they were able to overcome the crisis and enjoy the new family configuration of 4 members. Now, they deal with this new crisis, which seems incomprehensible to James, who feels sorry and sad for Margaret and keeps claiming that he is not interested in other women, that he is in love with his wife, and that he wants to spend the rest of his life with her. Margaret is not reassured by James's words: she is obsessed by the idea that he is cheating on her with Glenn. Also, going to the sports club has become difficult for the couple because of the misunderstandings regarding James's and Glenn's behaviours and the rumours about him that, according to Margaret, are circulating.

The therapist decides to see the clients individually, guided by the idea that some secrets could not be shared in the joint session. However, at the end of the individual sessions, she feels even more confused: James and Margaret told coherent stories, and they both looked sad and suffering for the on-going crisis; in other words, no differences emerged between individual and joint sessions.

The therapist formulated the hypothesis that Margaret's jealousy served to reconnect the couple, who was transiting to a new phase of their life cycle, namely the "empty nest", when children get older, autonomous, and ready to move out of the family household. The therapist shared with the couple this idea, and, surprisingly, they both agreed; however, they brought back the conversation to the present, to what Glenn did or did not do, and to their helpless frustration.

The therapist feels stuck and frustrated like the couple, and she begins to feel helpless. Both Margaret and James accepted the therapist's interpretation of jealously being what keeps them together; however, nothing has changed. How can the therapist make sense of the jealousy from a different perspective? The therapist reflects upon the fact the partners shared her hypothesis, but jealousy remains something negative for them; more precisely, it is the expression of an accusation made by Margaret to James.

In common sense, jealousy is an accusation whose opposite is defence; this dualism is projected onto the couples in terms of: "one accuses the other who defends him/herself from the accusation". These positions are two irreducibly opposite points of view. The therapist was about to get stuck in these rigid opposites. Margaret's and James's dualistic points of view could be overcome only through the adoption of a complementary perspective that connects the opposites: *How can Margaret's jealousy be seen as a form of defence/protection for James? But also, how can James's defence be seen as a way to reiterate his love for Margaret?*

The therapist reflects on the stage of the couple's transition: both partners were sports persons who started to realize that getting older means having fewer physical resources to continue to practice sports. In other words, they are facing the perspective of a physical and psychological decline, which is typical of older age. In this scenario, Margaret's jealousy undoubtedly causes discomfort to James, but from another point of view it helps him "cheer up" in a moment in which he feels older and depressed. In fact, Margaret's jealously is both the expression of an accusation of misbehaviour by James and a message to him about his desirability as a man to the extent that he could be attractive to a 20-year-old woman. In other words, jealously evokes the image of James as a still attractive man. On the other side, James's defence from Margaret's accusations confirms that despite being potentially attractive to a young woman, he continues to choose his wife. The therapist shares with the couple these reflections. James and Margaret are very impressed by the therapist's comment: Margaret nonverbally confirms it, and James exclaims: "Well, that's something big!"

Once the therapist overcame a rigid definition of jealously, she was more comfortable in exploring further aspects of the couple life. In fact, the subsequent sessions have focused on the clients' fear of getting older and their future as a couple and as individuals, helping them to cope with the sadness that resulted from the acceptance of their limitations. Both partners were invited to reflect on a new agreement as a couple regarding the new phase of their life as a couple, where they were able first to keep issues of jealousy and cheating out of the therapy and then out of their lives afterwards. Once again, Margaret and James were able to overcome the crisis and consolidate their relationship.

Deconstructing dominant beliefs

Research on social cognition has highlighted how social communities construct *social representations* of the phenomena they deal with; these forms of knowledge are believed to be real instead of just the constructions of the phenomena. Ideas are no longer perceived as products of social constructive processes, but as a reflection of something that exists outside [Farr and Moscovici 1984]. They are expressions of the dominant ideas that are universally taken for granted, conceived as natural phenomena and as such not questioned. Naturalized beliefs are shared and considered as "reality".

Several scholars have pointed out the potentially iatrogenic effects of this form of knowledge when psychotherapists unknowingly use it in therapy sessions. "Therapists may be unconscious of the extent to which their clinical decisions and theory choices are explained by their values. They need to examine the relationship between their values and their theoretical orientation because they may find themselves in a position where a given theory poorly accounts for certain client presentations" [Roysircar 2004, p. 660]. Therefore, in therapeutic settings it is essential to question shared beliefs and taken-for-granted dominant knowledge regarding a specific area of intervention, to deconstruct them, and to clear the context from potential denial of implicit prejudices. For instance, Byrne and McCarthy [1988] have argued that when working with families in which incest is revealed, it is important to consider the social representations of incest that may also be shared by therapists; this will prevent therapists from being trapped in loops of denial, imposition, control, and negative emotions. Pendry [2012] underlined how therapists who are unaware of the impact of race and racism upon the lives of their clients, would fall short in their capacity to assess, plan, and provide appropriate treatment. In psychological interventions with migrants, both prejudices and the notion of culture should be deconstructed; otherwise, these notions could unconsciously influence the efficacy of treatments in terms of co-construction and sharing of meanings [Rober and DeHaene 2014; Davolo and Fruggeri 2016]. Similarly, professionals working with chronic clients, for whom a network of services is involved, should reflect on the shared representations of the concepts of chronicity, network therapy, and rehabilitation [Fruggeri *et al.* 1995]. Over the last years, the transformations of families globally have required psychotherapists – not only family therapists – to reflect on how their representation of family, which often, unconsciously, overlaps with the idea of nuclear family, can drive them to adopt models that are inappropriate for providing counselling to clients belonging to non-traditional families [Singh 2009]. Furthermore, the development of assisted reproductive technologies has confronted professionals with their ideas of parenthood, maternity, and fertility [Grilli and Parisi 2016]. Therapists working with LGBT+ clients should consider the heterosexist culture that still characterizes many communities, agencies, and organizations [Everri *et al.* 2021]. Similarly, how can therapists work with women, depressed mothers, lonely wives, and marginalized young women without having deeply reflected on the myths regarding womanhood, maternity, the prescription of "sacredness and sacrifice", and all the moralistic expectations attached to the feminine gender role [McCarthy 2001]? It is only by challenging these conceptions that therapists can maintain a therapeutic position, like in the case presented below.

Vanessa is hospitalized for a relapse due to heroin addiction, after a long period of abstinence. She is 31 years old; she lives with her parents and her

2-and-a-half-year-old daughter, Rose. Vanessa's parents are both elderly and in poor health. Her older sister, Hillary, lives in the same town; she is married and has two young children. Hillary is an important support for Vanessa, who defines her as extremely reliable, maternal, socially committed, and "the exact opposite of her". Vanessa has done various jobs: waitress, factory worker, and shop assistant. Five years ago, she met Johnny, who was 4 years older than her and had been drug addicted for a long time. Vanessa moved in with him and started using cocaine and injecting heroin. After 3 years of cohabitation, Vanessa left Johnny and afterwards discovered she was pregnant. She decided to keep the baby, went back to live with her parents, and stopped using drugs. Vanessa told Johnny she was expecting a baby, but he said he was not interested in having a family. Rose, their baby girl, was given Vanessa's surname, and she looked after her with the support of her family and her sister. When Rose turned 7 months, Johnny contacted Vanessa claiming he wanted paternal rights to his daughter; Vanessa refused. Johnny threatened her and eventually started a legal battle for rights to Rose. The court denied the father's rights legitimation and issued a restraining order for Johnny, who was not allowed to see the mother and daughter. Johnny disappeared. Vanessa spent 2 good years in which she took care of her daughter and worked as a cleaner, until 6 months ago, when she had a relapse, and restarted using drugs frequently, spent all her savings, and had frequent conflicts with her family. Hillary, her sister, often had to intervene and take care of Rose because Vanessa was not going back home, and the grandparents were unable to mind the child. The situation became critical with the risk of a referral to social services when Vanessa decided to seek help in a service for drug addiction. She was hospitalized, and a rehab programme was developed for her. Rose was placed in the care of Hillary since the grandparents did not have the resources to look after the child without support. Vanessa followed the preparation to the rehab pro-gramme with strong motivation. She attended the meetings with her carers, nurses, and social workers, to plan together the subsequent steps of the pro-gramme. Hillary sometimes took Rose to meet Vanessa. However, as the time of being transferred to a rehabilitation community (where Vanessa was supposed to spend at least a year) was approaching, she became progressively more anxious and started showing concerning behaviour towards the social workers that they read as paranoid symptoms: Vanessa accused the professionals of wanting to remove the child from her care. Social workers on their part reassured Vanessa telling her: "Nobody wants to remove Rose's custody from you. At the moment, you are not capable of looking after her; you cannot have her now. You need to take care of yourself so that you can go back to your role as a mother at the end of the rehab programme". This message did not reassure Vanessa, who became increasingly anxious to the extent that the rehab team doubted she was ready to enter a programme for house residential treatment. The team asked for a supervision.

The supervisor invited the team to reflect on Vanessa's story, which was characterized by drugs use but also by efforts at being a mother. She showed she could be a "good mother": she detoxed when she became pregnant, she protected her daughter from the unrealistic requests of the biological father, and she took care of her daughter for 2 years. Vanessa had a relapse, which brought a series of negative consequences; however, she voluntarily decided to start a rehab programme. The situation was complicated since Vanessa is supposed to spend at least 1 year in a rehabilitation clinic to overcome drug use. Vanessa seems to ask the social workers the following question: "What will happen to my role as a mother while I am recovering?" The team answered to this question with: "You will get that role after you have recovered". The supervisor invited the team to reflect on the idea of motherhood underlying the conversation they had with Vanessa; she prompted the team to adopt a self-reflective position to deconstruct rigid conceptions and allow for the emergence of new ideas and solutions [see also Salamon and McCarthy 2016]. Both Vanessa and professionals shared the same idea of "intermittent motherhood", namely a role that could go on standby when Vanessa was taking care of herself. This generated a paradox with respect to Vanessa's identity, which can be phrased as follows: "In order to be a good mother, I need to recover and stay away from my daughter, but while I am away and take care of myself, I lose my role as a mother". This paradox derived neither from Vanessa's erroneous interpretation nor from the rehab team's lack of clarity in the conversations with her. Instead, the paradox is a logical consequence of a wrong premise: a mother is a good mother if she stays close to her children. This is a misleading conception of motherhood since it considers motherhood as presence not as a function, as a role not as a relationship. This conception is shared by both ordinary people and the mainstream scientific community[2]. Yet, a mother can be a good mother if she cares for the children's well-being and guarantees their protection, which does not necessarily depend on physical presence. Therapists working with women with psychological problems or drug addiction could acquire King Solomon's wisdom, who, as reported in the Bible, understood that renouncing maternal rights for the sake of the child was the best expression of motherhood (see Box 6.1). In other words, professionals should build upon a perspective that values the relationship. In so doing, they can create conversations that support the continuity of the mothers' identity while the women are recovering. Professionals need to deconstruct their assumptions of "good mother" to embrace a perspective that does not place the role of mother in opposition to her self-care. The coexistence of care for oneself with the role of mother is possible when the criterion of presence, intended as the foundation of motherhood, is replaced by the criterion of children's well-being. Starting from these reflections in the supervision session, the team decided to give Vanessa this message: "You don't have to worry about being your baby's mother. By separating from her to take care of yourself, you show how much you love her and care for her. In fact, you, as a good mother, accept staying away from your daughter, even though you suffer from the separation. By taking care of yourself, you allow her to enjoy a fully recovered mother". This message does not convey the idea that motherhood can live or be suspended *according to* different circumstances; rather, this stresses that a mother can continue to care for her daughter's well-being *across* different circumstances. This is a subtle and deep difference that can be practiced only after a process of deconstruction of the concept of motherhood as presence.

Box 6.1   King Solomon's wisdom

Then two prostitutes came to the king and stood before him. The one woman said, "Oh, my lord, this woman and I live in the same house, and I gave birth to a child while she was in the house. Then on the third day after I gave birth, this woman also gave birth. And we were alone. There was no one else with us in the house; only we two were in the house. And this woman's son died in the night because she lay on him. And she arose at midnight and took my son from beside me, while your servant slept, and laid him at her breast, and laid her dead son at my breast. When I rose in the morning to nurse my child, behold, he was dead. But when I looked at him closely in the morning, behold, he was not the child that I had borne." But the other woman said, "No, the living child is mine, and the dead child is yours." The first said, "No, the dead child is yours, and the living child is mine." Thus, they spoke before the king. Then the king said, "The one says, 'This is my son that is alive, and your son is dead'; and the other says, 'No; but your son is dead, and my son is the living one.'" And the king said, "Bring me a sword." So a sword was brought before the king. And the king said, "Divide the living child in two, and give half to the one and half to the other." Then the woman whose son was alive said to the king, because her heart yearned for her son, "Oh, my lord, give her the living child, and by no means put him to death." But the other said, "He shall be neither mine nor yours; divide him." Then the king answered and said, "Give the living child to the first woman, and by no means put him to death; she is his mother."

[First Book of Kings 3, 16–27]

Providing multiple descriptions of the same event

Meanings attributed to behaviours, events, and situations depend on the criteria used by social actors. In other words, any behaviour, event, or situation can have different meanings depending on the context in which it occurs and on the perspective taken to observe it. In this sense, a good exercise for practicing complex thinking is creating multiple descriptions of the same event. This allows therapists to overcome rigidity, embrace flexibility, and abandon explanations that are not useful to the therapeutic process. Consider the case example illustrated below.

Daniel is a young man aged 19 years who spent 1 year in a psychiatric rehabilitation centre. At the end of that period, he had fully recovered. In preparation for his formal discharge, the team suggested that he spend some days at home with his mother. Three days before the discharge from the psychiatric centre, Daniel asked to urgently talk to the psychiatrist since he had discovered that his mother was abusing alcohol. In light of this new information, the team wondered whether they should postpone Daniel's discharge. They decided to discuss the case in a supervision session. The supervisor invited the team to reflect on the following question: "What premise guides your concern about Daniel's discharge?". The team reported that Daniel had recently concluded a psychiatric rehab programme in which he was gradually acquiring self-confidence and autonomy. Asking him to look after his mother who was abusing alcohol would put excessive responsibility on him, thereby threatening the success of the rehab project. Some members of the team noticed the coincidence between Daniel's going back home and the mother's abuse of alcohol and interpreted this as a sign that the family was not ready yet for Daniel's return home. The rehab team's concern was understandable; however, this idea made them feel frustrated: they had to delay Daniel's discharge, thereby giving up the good outcome of their intervention. For this reason, they felt stuck. The supervisor suggested that the team's preoccupations might result from considering Daniel only as a psychiatric patient. The label of psychiatric patient often overshadow other characteristics of the person. When considering him a psychiatric patient, the professionals interpreted the communication with the psychiatrist as the expression of his vulnerability and his lack of capacity in dealing with a difficult situation. It may be there are other ways to define Daniel. The supervisor evoked the strand of studies on the Self and identity, which had shown how people express different parts of the Self according to different relational and dialogical contexts [Hermans 2002; Goncalves and Guilfoyle 2009]. Building upon this premise, the supervisor elaborated 2 questions that helped the team to embrace a different perspective on the case: "Which part of the Self did Daniel express in the conversation with the psychiatrist?" and "From what position was Daniel speaking when he reported his concern about his mother's behaviour?". These questions allowed the team members to observe this case from a different point of view: Daniel talked to the psychiatrist from the position of a son worried for his mother's health, and as such he was seeking help to manage a problematic situation. The decision to delay Daniel's discharge would have kept Daniel in the position of the psychiatric patient. Instead, acknowledging the position of son, the team could discharge him as planned, acknowledge his concern, and offer him support for looking after his mother. The follow-up of this case showed that Daniel was able to get the high school diploma, his mother followed a detox programme, and currently, they are both doing well.

The idea that different relational contexts activate different parts of the Self is particularly useful in situations in which a diagnosis is institutionally required. However, the diagnosis can become the filter through which every behaviour of the diagnosed person is interpreted. Cecchin claimed that the human being disappears behind the label [Boscolo *et al.* 1987, p. 43]. This can threaten the efficacy of the treatment since it introduces a rigid interpretation of the observed behaviours. The example described above clearly illustrates the importance of going beyond labels to embrace the idea that persons are complex and express themselves in different ways according to different contexts. Daniel was not only a psychiatric patient, but also a son concerned for his mother, a student who wanted to study for his high school diploma, a young man, etc. When the team started to shift their gaze and looked at the different parts of Self that Daniel expressed in different contexts, they became aware that what they interpreted as vulnerability could be seen as an adult son's sense of responsibility.

In some contexts, the actions of professionals put clients in rigid psycho-pathological roles, in which clients are always described in negative terms. Of course, a therapeutic intervention is provided when a problem or a critical situation prevents an individual from feeling well, evolving, and changing in a positive way. However, this obvious premise often risks activating a rigid and asymmetrical dynamic in which the client is the one who has the problem, and the therapist is the expert who must solve it.

In contrast to the context of psychiatric interventions, such a rigid dynamic is less likely to occur in counselling or psychotherapy; however, the risk of delivering interventions guided by psychopathological premises is always around the corner. Therefore, a paradoxical situation might emerge: therapists work to support clients to solve their problems, but they may adopt a perspective that prevents them from seeing a possible path of change and evolution. A perspective centred on psychopathology makes professionals see pathology. In other words, this is a rigid point of view that supports the interpretation of the psychological problems expressed by clients only in a negative way, thereby overshadowing resources and positive aspects. The case example below illustrates the need to overcome this perspective.

Vera is 27 years old and has a baby son, Julian, aged 1.5 years, with Tony, who is 30. They are both drug addicts. Since her pregnancy, Vera had started a detoxication programme, which she attended intermittently, while Tony continued taking drugs. Therefore, little Julian was placed in the grandparents' custody. Vera was able to finish the detoxication programme and went temporarily to live with her parents. The team planned to continue Vera's rehab programme in a mother–child residential home; Vera was initially happy with that, but as the date for moving in was approaching, she started feeling nervous and anxious. The professionals were unsure about their initial plan; therefore, they decided to ask for a supervision session.

Some members of the team interpreted Vera's anxiety as fear of taking responsibility for her child, since she had not spent much time with little Julian. They also considered that maybe she was not ready to be a mother; thus, it would have been better for her to start a rehab residential programme without Julian, who could have lived with his grandparents while Vera was away. This was a possible perspective on the case; however, it entailed looking at Vera's actions and reactions in her role as a patient. As in Vanessa's case described earlier, this view introduces the idea that the maternal role and the need to recover from addiction are incompatible.

A psychologist, a member of the team, proposed another interpretation: Vera's anxiety for going into a mother–child residential home derived from her role as a mother, since on the one hand she wanted to stay with Julian, and on the other hand, she was concerned about taking him with her to a rehab centre for drug addicts. This perspective implied changing the team's initial rehab programme and providing Vera with a rehab residential programme without the child; however, this would have had different implications for Vera's identity. Adopting this new perspective would have allowed them to see Vera's anxiety as willingness to protect her child from an environment that could have been seen as inappropriate, instead of her not being ready to be a mother. The team decided to have a conversation with Vera starting from this new premise. This allowed Vera to disclose other important concerns, which opened up other challenges and dilemmas about her future. She was unsure whether her parents would have taken Julian for the entire period of her rehabilitation. This aspect was not taken into consideration by the professionals, who then realized that they had to support Vera in negotiating Julian's care with her parents. Vera was not just a drug addict undertaking a rehab programme; she was also a mother who needed to find a way to take parental responsibility in a particularly complex situation. Furthermore, she was a daughter who had to negotiate the relationship with her parents in a situation in which she was moving from the role of the problematic daughter to the role of a daughter who became a mother and was asking her family's collaboration to be able to exercise her maternal role.

The attribution of positive intentions to others' behaviour is a way of getting disentangled from explanations that are not useful for both therapist and client. Therefore, taking a benevolent attitude can prevent therapists from providing rigid interpretations influenced by a pathological approach, which makes transformative solutions invisible. The idea that social actors can take different positions according to different contexts and circumstances is a useful tool to create different descriptions and interpretations of the same behaviour. The choice of descriptions or interpretations that can be useful should be based on the careful evaluation of what can foster interventions based on resources rather than on deficits.

Practicing divergent thinking

Another useful method for fostering complex thinking is practicing *divergent thinking*, namely seeking novelty instead of confirmation, identifying differences instead of sameness, and considering every situation as bringing something new and unexpected. Divergent thinking allows therapists to look at events and behaviours through a transformative therapeutic perspective, which is informed by a focus on micro-transitions rather than on change with a capital C. In such a perspective, therapists become able to observe and analyze interactive processes according to the small transformative events that occur during therapy rather than according to a desired final outcome. Divergent thinking is particularly useful for the treatment of psychiatric cases since the complexity and severity of symptoms can easily drive to chronicity. However, chronicity is not generated by the characteristic of the problem, but by the tendency to look for the confirmation of the problem, instead of enhancing the resources deriving from small changes for the time being (i.e., micro-transitions). Consider the next case example.

Mark is 27 years old and has a longstanding psychiatric history. He has spent more time of his life in psychiatric wards than at home. He showed aggressive behaviours against his family members: his mother, his father, his father's new wife, and his sister. Mark and his sister lived with their mother. The relationship between the 2 ex-spouses was very conflictual, especially when they talked about Mark. The mother wanted the father to look after Mark; the father accused his ex-wife of being the cause of Mark's problems, and when he offered to take Mark with him, Mark had an episode of acting out and ended up in the psychiatric ward. The referral documentation reports that the family had an interview with a family therapist, who at the end of the first and only session told the parents that Mark would never recover if they continued to quarrel in such a furious way.

Mark's aggressive behaviour became a serious problem also for the community in which the family lived. Both the family and the community became rejecting, and Mark continued to be hospitalized: the psychiatric ward progressively assumed the role of a caring family as opposed to the family of origin, which was excluding him. However, Mark's repeated hospitalizations made him a chronic patient who could no longer stay in a ward; therefore, the team decided to place him in a residential psychiatric centre. Mark continued to be a vulnerable patient. Every time he went out, accidents occurred: conflicts, assaults, and violent quarrels.

In this scenario, Mark's parents arrived at the residential centre stating that they wanted to take Mark with them to a town 900 kilometres away for an important family reunion that Mark could not miss. The team was astonished to hear that and tried to explain to the parents that it would have been quite risky to take their son on such a long journey as well as to attend a large family gathering. The parents, on their part, insisted they needed to take Mark with them and got very angry listening to the concerns of the team. After that meeting, both Mark's sister and the father's wife, contacted the team arguing for Mark's participation in the family reunion. The whole family was strongly in favour of having Mark with them; the professionals were scared about what might have happened.

In the supervision session, the team was invited to reflect on what was new in the request of the family. The team concurred that it was the first time that all family members shared the same idea and a project in which Mark was appearing good. In other words, it was the first time in which the family wanted Mark to be included instead of excluded. This was a completely different scenario, in which Mark could be expected to behave in a completely different way. The team decided to let him go, and things went very well. After this episode, the relationships among family members and between the family and the team changed dramatically to the extent that meetings with Mark and his family were planned to collaboratively work on a programme that allowed him to move into a supervised apartment, where he currently lives.

Divergent thinking that supports a transformative therapeutic perspective is crucial also in clinical cases that are at less risk of chronicity. It is always useful to adopt a transformative perspective that allows therapists to grasp the tiny signs of change and amplify them. As underlined by Boscolo and Bertrando [1994], each session brings a different story, the client (individual, couple, or family) in each session is an unedited entity. Lacking the individuation of potential changes across the therapy sessions might open the path to "endless therapies". When a therapist begins to see only redundant patterns or repetitions of dynamics, it is the time to change their point of view through the practice of divergent thinking.

Notes

1 Psychological problems of clients can derive from a dualistic conceptualization of complementary elements [Ugazio 2013]. However, in this chapter we want to stress that therapists can also share a dualistic epistemology, which does not allow them to help clients to overcome a rigid approach to the problem.
2 In a meta-analysis of the scientific literature [Visentini 2006] has identified 8 parental functions. The first function concerns the presence of the parent, which is defined by 5 dimensions: presence in the same household; presence that the child can see; presence that facilitates the interaction with the environment; presence in terms of interaction with the child; and presence as physical protection and security.

References

Bateson, G. [1979], *Mind and nature: a necessary unity*, New York, Bantam Books.
Batson, C.D., Duncan, B.D., Ackerman, P., Buckley, T. and Birch, K. [1981], *Is empathic emotion a source of altruistic motivation?*, in Journal of Personality and Social Psychology, 40, pp. 290–302.
Boscolo, L. and Bertrando P. [1994], *The times of time: a new perspective in systemic therapy and consultation*, London, W.W. Norton & Company.
Boscolo, L., Cecchin, G., Hoffman, L. and Penn, P. [1987], *Milan systemic family therapy*, New York, Basic Books.
Brown, B. [2015], *Rising strong*, New York, Penguin Random House.
Byrne, N. and McCarthy, I. [1988], *Moving statutes: re-questioning ambivalence through ambiguous discourse*, in The Irish Journal of Psychology, 9, pp. 173–182.
Davolo, A. and Fruggeri, L. [2016], *A systemic-dialogical perspective for dealing with cultural differences in psychotherapy*, in I. McCarthy and G. Simon (eds.), *Systemic therapy as transformative practice*, Farnhill UK, Everything Is Connected Press, pp. 111–124.
Everri, M., Mancini, T., Fruggeri, L. and O'Brian, V. [2021], *Cultivating practices of inclusion towards same-sex families in Italy: a comparison among educators, social workers, and healthcare professionals*, in Journal of Community & Applied Social Psychology, 31, pp. 659–672.
Farr, R. and Moscovici, S. (eds.) [1984], *Social representations*, Cambridge, Cambridge University Press.

Fruggeri, L. [1998], *Famiglie. Dinamiche interpersonali e processi psico-sociali*, Roma, Carocci.

Fruggeri, L., Marzari, M., Matteini, M. and Castellucci, A. [1995], *Servizi pubblici e terapia sistemica: teorie e tecniche nell'incontro con le famiglie*, in A. Gurman and D. Kniskern (eds.) *Manuale di terapia della famiglia*, Torino, Bollati Boringhieri, pp. 496–519.

Grilli, S. and Parisi, R. [2016]. *New family relationships: between bio-genetic and kinship rarefaction scenarios*, in Antropologia, 3, 1, pp. 29–51.

Gonçalves, M.M. and Guilfoyle, M. [2009], *Dialogism and psychotherapy: therapists' and clients' beliefs supporting monologism*, in Journal of Constructivist Psychology, 19, 3, pp. 251–271.

Hermans, H.J. [2002], *The dialogical self as a society of mind: introduction*, in Theory & Psychology, 12, 2, pp.147–160.

Keeney, B.P. [1983], *Aesthetics of change*, New York, Guilford Press.

Luyckx, K. and Vignoles, V.L. (eds.) [2012], *Handobook of identity theory and research*, NY, Springer.

McCarthy, I. [2001] *Fifth Province re-versings: 1 the social construction of women lone parents' inequality and poverty*, in Journal of Family Therapy, 23, pp. 253–277.

Pendry, N. [2012], *Race, racism and systemic supervision*, in Journal of Family Therapy, 34, pp. 403–418

Rober, P. and De Haene, L. [2014], *Intercultural therapy and the limitations of a cultural competency framework: about cultural differences, universalities and the unresolvable tensions between them*, in Journal of Family Therapy, 36, 1, pp. 3–20.

Roysircar, G. [2004], *Cultural self-awareness assessment: practice examples from psychology training*, in Professional Psychology: Research and Practice, 35, 6, pp. 658–666.

Salamon, E. and McCarthy, I. [2016], *Hope and risk: systemic practices for supervision and assessment in child protection*, in I. McCarthy and G. Simon (eds.), *Systemic therapy as transformative practice*, Farnhill UK, Everything Is Connected Press, pp 284–297.

Singh, R. [2009] *Constructing "the family" across culture*, in Journal of Family Therapy, 31, pp. 359–383.

Ugazio, V. [2013], *Semantic polarities and psychopathologies in the family: permitted and forbidden stories*, London, Routledge.

Varela, F. [1979], *Principles of biological autonomy*, New York, North Holland.

Visentini, G. [2006], Definizione e funzioni della genitorialità, available on the website http://www.genitorialita.it/documenti/le-funzioni-della-genitorialita/ (last accessed 10 giugno 2020).

7 Curiosity and decentring: distinguishing reasons from solutions

Curiosity, namely the interest in others' point of view, is another component – together with self-reflexivity and complex thinking – of therapists' epistemological competency, that is the ability to change points of view. In clinical practice, being curious means developing a deep interest in the lives of others and analysing their experiences within the context of their life stories. Therapists taking a position of curiosity encourage clients to tell stories that reveal their beliefs and their points of view, as well as to explore the ways in which they make sense of their lives. Also, curious therapists pose questions that invite the narration of stories otherwise hidden behind psychopathological descriptions. Furthermore, curiosity supports the exploration of clients' stories in a non-judgemental way, fosters the openness to different points of view, and allows therapists to support clients in amplifying the knowledge that clients have of themselves [Baptiste, Bellingar and Rachid 2019].

Cecchin's notion of curiosity [1987] derives from the assumption that it is vital for people to make sense of what they do, of others' behaviours, and of what is happening around them. Cecchin reiterated that people do not behave in a meaningless way. Some behaviours might appear meaningless to most; however, subjectively, there is always a reason, a context, and a point of view that help us make sense of people's actions. This perspective overturns the position of the observer: the idea that people have plausible reasons for what they do, shifts the attention from people's behaviours – even if incongruous and weird – to the reasons that are embedded in them. Consistently, the notion of curiosity is a second-order concept: it implies not only listening to the content of clients' stories but also developing an interest in the *ways people make sense of their experiences and choices*. This difference is paramount: therapists can either listen to their clients' stories from their points of view and their own premises, or they can reflect on how clients make sense of their own stories. When therapists listen from their own perspective, they might draw the conclusion that the clients' stories, the characters, and the described behaviours are wrong, senseless, or mad. Differently, when they reflect on clients' behaviours looking at their reasons, they could be able to understand that the clients' stories do, in fact, make sense. In Cecchin's terms, behaviours always happen within a context (defined as situation, relation, event, desire, need, etc.), which contributes to bring meaning to such behaviours

DOI: 10.4324/9781003278092-11

[Cecchin 1987]. Curious therapists should not look at the best or at the most logical explanation of a behaviour; they should rather adopt an aesthetic approach [Bateson 1979], which allows them to observe and understand *patterns,* namely ways in which thoughts, relations, and behaviours connect within the story of that person, in that specific system, in a given context.

Taking clients' perspective

The first requirement in practicing curiosity is to learn to decentre in order to "join" clients where they are. Decentring means moving away from one's own position to better understand things from the perspective of the clients. In so doing, therapists can avoid relying on premises – informed by scientific or common sense knowledge – that reify the clients' problem or colonize them and open instead a space for the expression of clients' subjectivity, thereby acknowledging them as competent interlocutors. As already discussed in the previous chapters of this book, psychotherapies aim at introducing differences and creating new stories that can be more useful for sustaining people's well-being. The notion of curiosity reminds us that newness can be created through a dialogical process that starts from "where" people are. Therapists introduce differences; they do not impose differences. In other words, they co-construct, together with clients, new stories in which clients' psychological and social needs can be rewritten within a new narrative script in which clients can find more suitable ways to respond to their own needs.

Curious therapists reflect on what works for clients instead of what does not work; also, they are interested in what connects stories, relationships, events, and positions even when they seem to be contradictory. In fact, apparently contrasting or senseless behaviours can make sense when a particular episode, a specific situation, or a personal experience is considered. As an example, people looking untidy and wearing filthy rags to the extent that they look like beasts in others' eyes, have often been victims of violence and abuse without being able to receive support or protection. Looking disgusting or nasty prevents people from being assaulted but also from receiving help. In this sense, such behaviours convey a double message: one's need to be protected and one's distrust in others being able to protect. Therefore, instead of talking about such behaviours (being dirty vs cleaning up, non-caring vs taking care of oneself, etc.), trust (that is the quality of the relationship) becomes the key topic in the conversations with clients showing such behaviours (see Box 7.1).

Box 7.1   The coprophagic boy

A 14-year-old boy with proven severe learning difficulties was interned in a state reformatory due to numerous delinquent behaviours (theft, dealing, drug use). After a period of poor adaptation to institutional life, the boy began to sprinkle himself with faeces and eat it. After several attempts at intervention, the professionals ask for supervision because they cannot understand whether that behaviour is due to intellectual disability or to a psychotic process. The supervisor asks the professionals a question typical of the systemic approach: "in which context would eating and spreading one's faeces on oneself be an appropriate behaviour for this boy?" An investigation conducted on the boy's story reveals that he had suffered sexual violence by other inmates in the institution. Obviously, since he had begun to cover himself with faeces and eat it, everyone avoided him: the coprophagia protected him from violence. But it was also a sign that he didn't trust the professionals of the institution to protect him. Having access to this understanding, the professionals oriented the intervention to reassuring the boy that they would protect him from further abuse [Cecchin, Lane and Ray 1992].

Decentring, namely understanding things from the point of view of clients, goes beyond the observed behaviour to grasp the meanings embedded in those behaviours. Some questions can favour decentring: in what context or from what point of view does this (the observed behaviour) make sense? What needs does this behaviour respond to?

These questions help therapists to develop a non-judgemental position and reach clients "where they are". From this position and through the connection with clients' feelings, emotions, and projects, therapists can help them to find new ways to reach their aspirations. This perspective introduces a crucial change in the ways therapeutic encounters are conducted: the focus is not on what is right or wrong, but on feelings, needs, and desires. In this sense, de-centring allows therapists to take a dialogical position that invites clients to participate in a relational process of shared meaning making. The case example below illustrates this dynamic.

Lilly is a young woman hospitalized in a ward that provides a first inter-vention leading to detoxification in the case of drug addiction, in preparation of the transfer to a rehab residential centre. The doctors thought that it was time for her to make this move, since Lilly showed a strong motivation to move forward and take care of herself. The nurses of the team, instead, argued she was not ready for a rehabilitation program: observing her behaviour during everyday life in the ward, they had noticed that she was seductive towards some visitors, and, recently, they caught her having sexual intercourse with other patients. In the nurses' opinion, these behaviours confirmed the idea that Lilly was not ready to undertake a rehabilitation programme. They thought she lied to doctors and did not really intend to take care of herself; otherwise, she would not have indulged in promiscuous behaviours. The team is torn between two positions: doctors thought Lilly was ready to move to the rehab centre; nurses thought she was not ready to cope with that program. The different points of view on the clinical case and the uncertainty about the best option for Lilly's treatment pushed the team to ask for a supervision session. Being aware that the question: "Who's right?" is useless, and the question "To whom did Lilly tell the truth?" cannot have an answer, the supervisor invited the team to decentre, to take a position of curiosity towards Lilly's point of view and feelings. More specifically, she suggested that the team replace their linear questions with other questions that looked at the meanings of Lilly's behaviours instead of their rightness. The questions were formulated as follows: "From what perspective does Lilly's behaviour make sense?" "What motivations might lead Lilly to present herself as a sexual object?" and "In what way can promiscuous sexual behaviour be seen as a way to take care of herself?" This type of question can favour decentring because it pushes the professionals to reconcile what seems irreconcilable. Building upon these initial reflections, the team was able to shift their attention from Lilly's behaviour to her desperate need to feel loved by someone. From this perspective, promiscuity assumed a new meaning; it could be conceived as an *inappropriate strategy* to achieve a *legitimate goal*. Indulging in promiscuous behaviour to satisfy the need for being loved was a shortcut that could have caused further suffering, and which could have prevented Lilly from achieving the goal of taking care of herself and being loved. This new perspective allowed the team to overcome the dualism in which they got stuck: Lilly intended to take care of herself as well as to go back to a "normal" life; the team had to support her to find a more functional strategy to reach that goal as well as to cope with the time required to complete the rehab programme.

The professionals' ability to change their points of view allowed them to see what held together apparently irreconcilable stories and positions. Promiscuity was inconsistent with undertaking a rehabilitation programme; however, promiscuity was consistent with the desperate desire to be loved by someone. Through the change of perspective solicited by the supervisor, Lilly no longer appeared as a liar; instead, she appeared as a distressed young woman. The members of the ward team (doctors and nurses) no longer felt they had to "correct" Lilly's inappropriate behaviours; rather, they felt they were therapists who had to help a young woman to continue with the recovery process without looking for shortcuts but enduring for the fulfilment of her needs.

The team reflections were shared with Lilly: they told her they understood her desire to improve her life as well as her need to be loved; yet, they wondered to what extent offering herself as a sexual object during the hospitalization was a useful way for achieving her goals. They clearly expressed concern about the shortcut of promiscuity since it was a way to distract her from her goals. Thanks to this type of conversation, Lilly could share with the professionals her fears both in terms of not being loved and of not being able to cope with the rehabilitation program. This gave the professionals the opportunity to offer her help to cope with the waiting time that the rehab process required.

Before the supervision session, the team had focused only on the goal of treatment, that is, on the transition to the rehab centre; consequently, they addressed their attention to Lilly's dysfunctional behaviours, thereby seeing them as inconsistent with the purposes declared by the young woman. Of course one could say that taking care of oneself and promiscuity are inconsistent behaviours; however, the notion of curiosity implies that even inconsistent behaviours must have a meaning. In other words, curiosity prompts psychotherapists to embrace a "therapeutic bias"; that is, clients' behaviours are connected to their psychological needs. In Gail Simon's words [2010, p. 315], therapists believe that "people are not 'bad' or 'inadequate', they are not 'difficult' or 'resistant', but they are acting out of self-preservation until the relational context is safe enough for them to emerge with confidence". This prejudice allows therapists to become curious and to look at things from the points of view of the clients, thereby being able to grasp the legitimate needs that clients bring to the therapeutic context. In so doing, therapists can move from a judgemental to a listening position, from which they can accompany clients in the achievement of their goals while safeguarding their well-being.

Legitimizing reasons and changing solutions

The development of curiosity towards clients' perspective is facilitated by the ability to separate the reasons from the solutions, or the goals from the strategies adopted to pursue them. People may have good reasons for doing something; yet, they may adopt solutions that are dysfunctional; similarly, people can have legitimate purposes, but they try to achieve them using inadequate strategies. Good reasons include: desires (for example, being loved), needs (for example, feeling protected), and moral duties (for example, helping those in need). Solutions can be more or less dysfunctional, and strategies can be more or less inadequate according to the impact they have on clients' lives, not according to the judgement of the therapist. Continuing with the case example described earlier, filling an emotional void with promiscuity is an inadequate strategy as long as promiscuous and casual sex does not bring love or affection. Reasons and goals should be kept separate from solutions and strategies since reasons/goals can be understood and legitimized, whereas solutions/strategies can be changed and made more appropriate to the goal. Focusing only on solutions and strategies inevitably leads to taking a judgemental position, deciding what is right and what is wrong in the client's behaviour. This also entails taking an "expert position" in which therapists delude themselves into thinking they know more than their clients do and that they can make decisions on their behalf. Instead, curiosity helps to overcome this position and develops an interest for the reasons/goals of clients, which should be legitimized to create a dialogical space for finding more functional solutions/strategies. In other words, the legitimization of clients' reasons/goals should not be overshadowed by the different ways in which they choose to pursue their goals.

The case example illustrated below shows that the reasons why clients use inappropriate strategies can be found in their life stories: clients may have had only that solution available at that time in their life. This can happen in situations in which social relations are limited, as described in the following case example [reported in Fruggeri and Matteini 1994].

Anne is a single mother living with Mark, her 7-year-old son. She has suffered from depression and has had negative experiences with men. She recently moved into a new city, where she found a job as a cleaner. She contacted social services since she needed to go to work every day at 8:00 am, including Saturdays, and was unable to look after her child because schools were closed on Saturdays. The social worker found a young woman, a university student, who volunteered to mind Mark, but Anne refused the proposed solution. Anne claimed she wanted a man to mind her son since she was a single mother and Mark would have benefited from having a male rather than a female figure as minder. The social worker in charge of the case was reluctant to accept this request, but eventually she managed to find a young man as a minder. However, Anne refused again, this time claiming she had already found a child minder for Mark; therefore, she was asking the social worker to pay him for his work. The social worker found such a request unacceptable and brought the case to the weekly supervision team meeting. The immediate reaction of the team was to judge Anne and consider her to be someone who wanted to exploit and manipulate the service. The supervisor invited the team to be curious about Anne's "good reasons" for making those requests. The team formulated the hypothesis that Anne felt lonely and wanted the support of a man for herself as a woman as well as for her child as a parent. From this perspective, Anne's requests could be seen as a plausible solution for both her problems: the loneliness of a single woman and the need of someone who could mind her son while she was at work. Nevertheless, Anne's solution was unacceptable to the social workers team as long as they did not have a budget for baby-sitting; however, her reasons were legitimate. The social worker shared the hypothesis formulated during the supervision session with Anne: she discussed with her whether the man she was looking for was an actual support or the recipient of hopes and expectations that could hardly be attended. Also, it was proposed to deal with her problems separately, namely accept that the student could take her child to school and mind him while she was at work, and she could talk to someone about her loneliness to explore possible solutions.

Anne's case example clearly shows that the focus on the solutions that Anne proposed was driving the social work team towards a judgemental position that was marginalizing the client. This not only brought the risk of the service failing with Anne (yet another failure for Anne!), but also a sense of frustration and helplessness for the social workers. Instead, focusing on Anne's reasons and the meanings of her requests allowed the social worker to engage in a dialogue in which Anne's needs could be acknowledged and the team could provide a form of support that was co-constructed and not imposed.

Clients finding dysfunctional solutions to a problem are not necessarily suffering situations of poverty, of social disadvantage, or of pathology; they may be guided by values or moral duties to find solutions that prove inadequate for their well-being. Lucy's case exemplifies how a young woman was willing to sacrifice herself for her mother's sake.

Lucy is a 24-year-old woman who is close to graduating with a degree in architecture. She lives with her parents, both in their 50s: her father works as an employee in a bank, while her mother is a teacher. Lucy has an older brother who works in the IT sector and lives with his partner. Lucy decided to start psychotherapy during a period of personal crisis: she felt sad and un-motivated in different areas of her life. She has always been a good student and has wanted to become an architect since she was a child; however, over the last year she had problems with concentration and studying for her exams.

Lucy is not happy with her relationships: she had a boyfriend for 2 years after she finished high school, but since then she has only had occasional dates. She wants to find a man to love and live with, but she thinks men do not like her. She has had 2 good friends since she was a child, but they started to hang out with a group of college friends that she does not know. Lastly, she defines her family as an "apparently normal family" since her mother has an addiction to alcohol, but neither her mother nor her father have ever acknowledged the problem. Lucy says her mother habitually drinks every evening and sometimes also during the day; on weekends, she drinks more than usual. However, nobody has addressed the problem so far.

Lucy and her father look after her mother: they make sure she is not alone in the evening, and they drive her to school meetings so that she cannot stay in bars; they fear that when she is drinking she could cause harm to herself and others. The mother has never had accidents, only because Lucy and her father monitor her closely and constantly. Lucy's brother has never been involved in the mother's care since he does not live at home.

The therapist starts the session building upon this background information and decides to explore what prevents Lucy from continuing to achieve her goals in the different realms of her life, namely attending college, having friends, and looking for a partner. Lucy explains that her family needs her help. She suffers because she wonders about what is going to happen to her in the future. She has nearly finished the exams, but once she is graduated, what can she do? Can she find a job as an architect? How far from home? For how many working hours? She enjoys hanging out with her friends and meeting people, but she feels she is different from her friends, who apparently do not have problems with their families. When she goes to the pub with her friends, she must check her phone often to make sure her father is back home on time, and when he is not, she must decide whether to leave and give up the night out or stay but without enjoying the company because of the concern for her mother.

The therapist asks Lucy what would happen if she stopped looking after her mother. Lucy says she cannot do that since her biggest concern is that her mother could harm herself while being drunk. The therapist wonders how she can help Lucy to escape the cage she is trapped in. But this idea proves to be useless, because Lucy reiterates that she must help the family to cope with her mother's addiction. To the therapist's eyes, Lucy was like a victim devoted to sacrifice. Her choice appeared senseless to the therapist, who instead thought that she should leave her mother to her father and dedicate her time to building her future. But, when therapists start thinking that clients' behaviour is senseless, it is the moment for them to become curious and start decentring by asking themselves: from what point of view does Lucy's choice make sense even if it gives her pain? Lucy feels that her mother's health and the family well-being depend on her; helping her family is a moral duty, and she cannot escape this situation. Clearly, the therapist's idea of "escaping" is not an option for Lucy. She is absolutely convinced that her family needs her support since the mother is not able to take care of herself and the father is unable to look after his wife alone; consequently, it is her duty to help, and the only way to help is to sacrifice her life. So, the therapist realizes that she cannot ask Lucy to give up what she feels is a moral duty; she cannot ask her to stop helping her family. Yet, she could suggest exploring the chance to find a more functional way to do it. The solution of sacrifice originates from a dichotomy: either I help my family, or I live my life. But the therapist is also trapped in the same dichotomy, thinking that Lucy could follow her life only by leaving her family. Is it possible for Lucy to help her family and at the same time live her life? How can these two aspects coexist? For supporting her mother and her father, Lucy needs to be well and to be happy with the choices she makes both in her personal and professional life. Being trapped in such a dichotomy, instead, can lead Lucy to need support herself in the long run.

After sharing these reflections, Lucy and the therapist continue exploring her possibilities of actions while remaining a support for her family. Lucy finally decides to talk to her father to acknowledge mother's problem and find professional help to support her dealing with her alcohol problem.

Looking for the client's reasons/goals helps therapists to take the client's perspective and connect with the client's feelings, emotions, desires, and plans, to find new and more functional ways to pursue them. As illustrated by Lucy's case example, understanding the client's perspectives means being able to explore and value new meanings that can be very different from those of the therapist.

Decentring from "white" ways of knowing

The importance of going beyond the behaviours, i.e., the dysfunctional solutions or strategies that people adopt, in order to reach people's deep reasons and needs is a fundamental methodological principle for those who work with clients belonging to different ethnic groups and especially with those who experience oppression and institutional violence. In these cases, understanding the client's perspective might entail the exploration of meanings that are culturally different from those of the therapists, who must then suspend their understanding and become curious about the client's understanding of their life experiences. The story of Fatna and her family is an example[1].

Fatna, 28, and Idriss, 34, are married. They arrived in Italy from an African country involved in a civil war. They have two children: Susheta, a girl of 6 years, and Hassan, a boy of 1 year, born in Europe. Fatna contacted the

Health Centre for Immigrants (HCI), showing a court order imposing the separation of the children from their parents. The reason for the order was that Fatna, while pregnant of her second child, had interrupted her participation in the Refugees Protection Programme, escaping abroad with Susheta. In the European country to which she had escaped, Fatna gave birth to Hassan. Few months later, the local authorities communicated to Fatna that, according to the Dublin Regulation, she and her children had to go back to Italy, the country in which she had started the procedure for asylum. Fatna returned to Italy and dutifully contacted the local police. The sudden and inexplicable departure of Fatna with Susheta, and her determination to avoid any explanation, worried the court to the point of ordering the social services to host Fatna and her children in a shelter while observing and supporting Fatna's parental skills. Meanwhile, Idriss was living with friends. While at the shelter, Fatna proved to be an adequate mother to her children; yet, she attempted to leave twice. For this reason, the court decreed that the children should be separated from their parents and demanded an assessment of Fatna's and Idriss' personalities. It is at this point that Fatna got in touch with HCI seeking help. During the consultation with the psychologist, Fatna appeared not to realize how potentially dangerous the situation was for her children. She minimized the episodes, gave incoherent explanations for her decisions, rejected any responsibility, and attributed a deliberate intention to harm her by the social workers. The situation appeared incomprehensible to the psychologist, who wondered, "Why does Fatna persist in running away from situations that are thought to be protective for her and her family?" Taking a curious position, this question was reframed as, "From which viewpoint is escaping from the Refugees Protection Programme a way for Fatna to protect her children?" Both questions are centred on the shared value that children need to be protected. But the first one implies that there is only one way to protect: that of the dominant culture (the social services, the Refugees Programme, the court). The second question implies that there are different ways to protect, and that Fatna was protecting her children according to assumptions of which the professionals were ignorant. With this question in mind, the therapist invited both partners for a meeting, during which the story of their family, the reasons of their migrating, and their hopes and fears could be explored.

After marriage, Fatna and Idriss escaped from their country because the government persecuted them. Fatna had to hide from a totalitarian state since her childhood: many of her relatives had been tortured and killed by the police. In the African country where they moved, they could live a quiet life for some years. Little Susheta was born there. The blow up of a new war forced them to escape once more. They arrived in Italy and were included in the Refugees Protection Programme. As refugees, they had to refer to Social Services for any needs. Yet, Fatna and Idriss were obsessed by the amount of time that the procedure for their asylum was taking. Since they didn't have a residency permit, they couldn't work. In the face of Fatna's second pregnancy, they wondered with worry how they could rear two children without working.

At this point of the session, the therapist asked, "What happens in your village at home when parents cannot raise their children?" Idriss answered that the parents would entrust their children to a member of the larger clan chosen by the elders in the father's family. So, the conversation continued:

Therapist: *Do you have relatives in Italy?*
Fatna: *No.*
Therapist: *So … the children …*
Idriss: *Children here belong to the State.*
Therapist: *What do you mean?*
Idriss: *If you don't have a job, Social Services decides.*
Therapist: *Did the social worker tell you this?*
Fatna: *No, a mediator told us that it could happen.*

This is how Idriss and Fatna made sense of the situation and acted accordingly. They had interpreted the meetings with the social worker as "warnings" that, in case they didn't prove to be able to solve their problems, the children would have been taken away. To avoid this, Fatna escaped. When she was sent back to Italy, she forcedly had to contact the police authorities, which in her experience are not seen as reliable since, in her life to date, she always had to escape from state authorities. After her placement, with her children, in the shelter, Fatna started to think that the social services were deliberately planning to harm her and her family. This piece of conversation highlighted two "blind spots" that prevented the development of a shared vision in the relationship between Fatna and the professionals. For the parents, *"the children of troubled parents belong to the clan"* translated in the migratory context as *"the children of troubled parents belong to the state"*, which for Fatna assumed a tragic meaning since for her *"the state is a prosecutor."* On the other side, the professionals assumed that *"a meaningless behaviour is a symptom"* and *"a mother who exposes her children to risky situations, cannot be a good mother."* These parallel visions acted in a self-referential way in this situation, yet confirming each other, thus generating a recursive spiral headed toward the worst outcome. The curiosity of the psychologist toward Fatna's viewpoint led to an understanding of all enacted behaviours. He then wrote to the social worker in charge of the case and offered his interconnected description of the situation, suggesting that she work with the couple in a way that possibilities might emerge for a third shared perspective from which it would be possible to co-construct Idriss and Fatna's "parenting in a context of forced migration."

The different facets of epistemological competency

Curiosity and decentring are key components of epistemological competency.

However, readers will have noticed that self-reflexivity, complex thinking, and curiosity are mutually connected in a recursive way. More specifically, curiosity prompts therapists to position themselves from the point of view of clients through reflection on the legitimate reasons that have guided their behaviours. Nevertheless, this is possible only when therapists practice self-reflexivity, which allows them to become aware of their blind spots to the reasons of clients, i.e., "naturalized" dominant ideas, implicit thoughts, personal beliefs, hidden prejudices, emotional problems, and social positioning. The focus on therapists' premises and positioning is paramount since it is a necessary condition for making therapists aware of the rigid interpretations that can emerge during the treatment and that can prevent them from approaching the points of view of their clients.

Decentring in order to grasp the perspective of other people requires therapists to distance themselves from their certainties and their truths; this can be possible when they practice complex thinking. Complex thinking means looking for differences and deconstructing common sense in order to create multiple descriptions of the same phenomenon and connect elements that appear as opposites. In fact, the reasons/goals of others can be understood and legitimized when therapists take an epistemological position from which they can acknowledge that different truths are possible. Therapists are committed to taking these epistemological positions since they are aware of psychotherapy not being a unilateral action. Decentring is also a way to reflect on how clients see therapists and thus on how clients make sense of therapy. As discussed in this and in the previous chapters, psychotherapy's outcome is always the result of a joint action in which clients participate with their premises, opinions, points of view, social status, cultural belongings, etc., which can be accessed by therapists through developing a dialogue from a position of curiosity.

Note

1 We thank our colleagues Andrea Davolo, Imelda McCarthy, and Gail Simon for authorizing the use of this case, whose expanded version is contained in [Davolo, A., and Fruggeri, L. 2016], *A systemic-dialogical perspective for dealing with cultural differences in psychotherapy*, in I. McCarthy and G. Simon (eds.), *Systemic therapy as transformative practice*, Farnhill UK, Everything is Connected Press, pp. 111–124.

References

Baptiste, D., Bellingar, K. and Rachid, I. [2019], *Curiosity in couple and family therapy*, in K. Lebow, A. Chambers and D. Breunlin (eds.), *Encyclopedia of couple and family therapy*, J, Switzerland, Springer.

Bateson, G. [1979], *Mind and nature: a necessary unity*, New York, Bantam Books.

Cecchin, G. [1987], *Hypothesizing, circularity, and neutrality revisited: an invitation to curiosity*, in Family Process, 26, 4, pp. 405–413.

Cecchin, G., Lane, G. and Ray, W.A. [1992], *Irreverence: a strategy for therapists' survival*, London, Karnac Books.

Davolo, A. and Fruggeri, L. [2016], *A systemic-dialogical perspective for dealing with cultural differences in psychotherapy*, in I. McCarthy and G. Simon (eds.), *Systemic therapy as transformative practice*, Farnhill UK, Everything is Connected Press, pp. 111–124.

Fruggeri, L. and Matteini M. [1994], *Poverty and social services*, in Human Systems, 5, pp. 319–336.

Simon, G. [2010], *Self-supervision, surveillance and transgression*, in Journal of Family Therapy, 32, pp. 308–325.

Part IV

Acknowledging the context: the social dimension of psychotherapy

8 Relational interdependence and triadic co-evolution

The wider context of psychotherapy

Bateson writes, "Without identification of context, nothing can be understood. The observed action is utterly meaningless until it is classified as 'play', 'manipulation', or what not" [1975, p. 147]. The context, as he pointed out, is the matrix of meanings [1972]. With this definition, this author provides a fundamental methodological indication that the systemic approach has taken as the foundation of its clinical model: no fact can be explained without considering the intertwining of present and past circumstances within which this fact emerges and develops. In this sense, therapists take into consideration the context within which symptomatic behaviours develop and are maintained, but also the context in which the manifestations of psychological suffering can dissolve, that is, the context of psychotherapy. A psychotherapeutic intervention does not take place in a vacuum, but within the intertwining of systems of meaning and interactions that characterize the clients' relationships within their environment [Rober 2017].

From this point of view, "acknowledging the context" concerns the therapist's awareness of operating in a broad environment, which goes beyond the therapy room, as long as clients have a life of their own out there, a life of relationships. Psychotherapy is not only a significant event for those who participate personally, but also, directly or indirectly, for those with whom clients have meaningful relationships. Whether it is an individual, a couple, or a family, what they experience in the encounter with the psychotherapist, what they feel, the results they achieve, the changes or non-changes they make, reverberate in their daily lives and in the network of relationships they belong to. Significant people with whom clients are in relationship participate through conversations – or even silences – about therapy, through observation of the relative's behaviour, and through commenting on some differences in behaviours or attitudes. Psychotherapy, whether the therapist is aware of it or not, is embedded in a network of interconnected systems, which affect and are affected by whatever occurs in the therapeutic process. As most psychotherapists know, for example, a significant improvement for a client involves a change for the whole family. Couple therapy that helps partners renegotiate their relationship may involve the

DOI: 10.4324/9781003278092-13

need to redefine the relationship with their families of origin as well. But sometimes the clients themselves bring their loyalties into the therapy rooms. The following excerpt from a patient's diary is a vivid example of what such loyalty can entail.

> I would not always overcome my exasperation. But even then, I was frequently influenced by a spirit of bravado and defiance of the doctors, to whom I knew my letters were subjected for inspection; I was determined, if they declared that my anger at being confined, and at my treatment, was a proof of my madness, that they should have evidence enough of it ... Even a deeper motive lay hid under all this violence of expression; and this may perhaps by many be deemed an insane motive: I knew that, of all the torments to which the mind is subject, there is none so shocking, so horrid to be endured as that of remorse for having injured or neglected those who deserved our esteem and consideration. I felt for my sisters, my brothers, and my mother: I knew they could not endure to look upon what they had done towards me, to whom they were once so attached, if they rightly understood it; that they could know no relief from the agony of that repentance which comes too late, gnawing the very vitals, but in believing me partly unworthy of their affection; and therefore I often gave the reins to my pen, that they might hereafter be able to justify themselves, saying he has forfeited our respect, he has thrown aside the regard due to his parentage and to his kindred – he has deserved our contempt, and merited our abandonment of him.
>
> [John Perceval's *Narrative of the treatment experienced by a gentleman,* 1840 reported in Bateson 1961, p. 49]

Professionals working with children who are victims of neglect on the part of their parents know the conflicting feelings the children have towards their parents. A therapeutic intervention conceived as an alternative to the family dysfunctional context is often rendered ineffective precisely by those who, in the professional intention, should be "saved" [Fruggeri 1998]. Whenever therapists take on the need of an individual client without considering the relational context within which this need is expressed, they run the risk of implementing behaviours that, for the client, may constitute a solution to the client's problems, but at the expense of some significant ties in the client's network of relationships. In this way, a relational situation is activated in which no one can establish an "alliance" with a significant other (the therapist) without this entailing at the same time a "counter-alliance" with another equally significant person (partner, parents, children). This is an interactive dynamic known as "loyalty conflict", which is dysfunctional for the development of the people involved.

All this considered, it can be said that the context of psychotherapy, be it individual, couple, or family, is always a triadic context: therapist, clients, and significant others. In this sense, "acknowledging the context" means equipping oneself with constructs that are useful to describe the triadic dynamics involved in every psychotherapeutic intervention.

The interdependence of relational contexts and their co-evolution

A therapeutic intervention does not take place in a temporal and contextual vacuum. Clients do not begin to exist at the moment they meet a therapist. They have a history, are involved in a network of relationships, and live with a number of bonds that define their belonging and therefore their identity. This composite framework constitutes the context of the therapeutic intervention, its matrix of meanings. A psychotherapist can grasp the impact of their actions in their clients' lives, when they adopt a model that has the interdependence of interactive-relational contexts as its organizing principle. That is, a model that highlights the triadic and circular nature of the processes that originate with the initiation of psychotherapy. The events that occur within the relationship between a therapist and a client trigger processes in the context of the re-lationship between the latter and his/her significant system, which in turn affect the evolution of the process that takes shape in the interaction between client and therapist. This is the principle of *relational interdependence* according to which the relationship between two people is never independent of the relationships that each of them entertains with significant others.

Furthermore, following the developmental psychologist Bronfenbrenner, we can affirm that the relationship between two people is evolutionary to the extent that it has positive repercussions on the relational contexts in which each is involved.

> The capacity of a dyad to function effectively as a context of development depends on the existence and nature of other dyadic relationships with third parties. The developmental potential of the original dyad is enhanced to the extent that each of these external dyads involves mutually positive feelings and the third parties are supportive of the developmental activities carried on in the original dyad. Conversely, the developmental potential of the dyad is impaired to the extent that each of the external dyads involves mutual antagonism or the third parties discourage or interfere with the developmental activities carried on in the original dyad.
> [Bronfenbrenner 1979, p. 77]

Finally, according to the principle of *co-evolution of systems*, a change in the quality and definition of the relationship between 2 individuals involves a change in the quality and definition of the relationships that each of them entertains with others and in the quality of the identities of everyone involved. In this perspective, "acknowledging the context" is a competency that is based on a model that we can define as co-evolutionary, which guides therapists: 1) to reflect on the meaning that their interventions with a client take on within the context of relationships between the client and his/her significant ones; and 2) to organize the intervention based on what they believe useful and evolutionary for the client as a component of a broader relational system and, therefore, useful and evolutionary for the whole system. Let's reflect on the following case.

Angie is 35 years old. She is divorced and has a daughter, Miriam, aged 8, and a son, Mark, aged 5. Three years ago, her ex-husband moved to another part of the country, and, after 2 years of sporadic visits, he broke off any contact. She is in treatment at the Mental Health Service for a depression that has greatly incapacitated her in the last 2 years: she left her job and had long periods of social withdrawal. Due to Angie's frequent hospitalizations, the children were entrusted to their maternal grandmother. Upon discharge from the last hospitalization, the professionals of the Mental Health Service suggest that Angie attend a day hospital so that she can carry out some activities, socialize with other guests, and participate in group therapy meetings. After a few months, she shows a visible improvement, to the point that the child protection social worker proposes to start operating so that Angie and her children can reconnect. For this purpose, they organize meetings between Angie and her children, during which they can spend time together.

The grandmother begins to complain and asks to meet the social worker to tell her about the difficulties that Miriam and Mark have shown since they have been meeting their mother. The grandmother says plainly that Angie has a bad influence on her children. She often calls her other daughter, Melanie, who lives in another city, expressing her concern for the grandchildren. Melanie, constantly urged by her mother, also asks to speak to the social worker and confirms her mother's version, stressing that Miriam and Mark need to continue to be with their grandma. The children, in this psychological climate, appear anxious when they attend the meetings with Angie, who in turn shows more and more tension when the day of the meeting with the children approaches. Finally, Angie has a very serious depressive crisis, locks herself up at home, does not want to see anyone, and, once more, is hospitalized in the psychiatric unit.

What happened? The professionals acted by limiting their vision to Angie's recovery process, without considering what a positive outcome of such process could have entailed in terms of redefining relationships, roles, and identities of all the people who are involved in Angie's context: if the meetings between Angie and the children had proved that she was able to manage the children, they could have returned to live with her. The grandmother would have then lost her role, found herself alone, and turned to her daughter, Melanie, who, in fact, was receiving increasingly pressing requests for care from her mother. Faced with these potential feared changes, the people involved enacted defensive behaviours to maintain their positions – behaviours, however, that repositioned Angie as the psychiatric patient unable to care for her children.

Angie's crisis signalled this. As Bronfenbrenner taught us, it was impossible for Angie to evolve positively without this entailing a positive evolution for others as well. Having acknowledged this, the professionals review their program of intervention, not in its aims, but in its process. To be guided, in fact, by the principles of relational interdependence and co-evolution does not mean giving up programs aimed at the recovery of client; it means doing it in a way that considers the reasons and needs of others, and therefore positioning them within the process as well. After this reflection, the professionals confirm the goal of reconnecting the relationships between Angie and the children, but involving the grandmother in the program, asking her to help this re-unification, and identifying the role that she would still maintain after the children have returned to live with mom. After being discharged from the Psychiatric Unit, Angie resumed attending the day hospital, and meeting with the children accompanied by grandmother, until she reached a new equilibrium in which her mother was available to support Angie's maternal role, taking care of the children when she went to the work that the Mental Health Service had provided for her in collaboration with a cooperative that deals with job placement as a therapeutic program.

Favouring personal independence by caring belonging

Families are interdependent systems, so much so that even a single member's transition requires the redefinition of everyone else's roles and relationships. For this reason, family therapy constitutes an elective intervention to help families who have difficulties in redefining roles, boundaries, relationships, and hierarchies in order to support the individual development of their members. However, in this respect, the transition of children to adult life appears to be particularly complex. On the one hand, children's entry into adulthood entails a redefinition of the couple relationship between the parents; therefore, family therapy could be appropriate. On the other hand, given that the core of the request for help is the personal independence of a young adult, individual therapy would be more appropriate, since the therapeutic setting would be a first assertion of the redefinition of the boundaries with respect to his/her parents.

Faced with a scenario of this type, therapists would show lack of understanding of the dynamics and processes involved in the client's life if they organize the intervention and evaluate its effects only in the context of their dyadic relationship with the client. In the specific case of individual therapy with a young adult, it would not be simply a matter of understanding whether and to what extent the presented difficulties are connected to issues in the family context. It would also be the case of applying the principle of co-evolution and evaluating how the emancipation of the child could reverberate in the parallel and interconnected process of redefining the relationship between parents. *The principle of co-evolution does not concern the origin of discomfort,* but *the effect that the resolution of discomfort could have on the client's relational context.* This does not mean abandoning the goal of helping the client; it rather means achieving such goal through a process that transforms the positive personal evolution into a positive evolution for everyone affectively connected. The following case is an example.

Following the advice of her general practitioner, Patricia contacts a psychotherapist for her 20-year-old son, Malcom. For a year now, Malcom has suffered from strange stomach aches that occur now and then and do not seem to be connected to any physical cause. Malcom saw several specialists (gastroenterologist, internist), but nothing significant emerged, so much so that the general practitioner suggested psychological treatment. Malcom is a brilliant young man, a music talent recognized both locally and nationally; he plays the violin, and after finishing high school, he started at the conservatory with excellent results. He is Patricia and Rendal's only child and lives with his parents. Before getting sick, he used to play sports, but it was during a fencing training that he began to feel the first abdomen pains, and from there on he has gradually withdrawn from his sports commitments until he stopped for good. During the last year, he has always met his tasks at the conservatory, albeit with great difficulty; he has managed to respect the concerts dates, but he has felt unwell several times, and on those occasions, he called his mother, who reached him to reassure and support him until the performance was over. When he is at home, he can play and concentrate for many hours, and if the stomach aches arrive, he can resist more than when he is away.

Patricia provides this information to the therapist, underlining that she is very worried about her son, above all because in recent months the situation has worsened to the point of her having to drive Malcom to the emergency room twice. The therapist asks if Malcom is aware of the phone call and if he agrees to start therapy. Patricia answers that he is right there beside her, listening to the phone call; Malcom did not call because usually she is the one who takes care of his health. The therapist decides to see Malcom alone for an initial consultation and asks Patricia to tell him to call her to make an appointment.

After a couple of days, Malcom calls and with a trembling voice asks to schedule an interview. Despite the first telephone contact, Malcom seems to be at ease in talking about himself, sharing his thoughts, emotions, and moods with the therapist. Malcom attends the sessions regularly, shows commitment and willingness to reflect on himself and his life. He is aware that he has become a bit isolated in the last year. Lately, he has not gone out with friends as he used to, and he has dedicated all his time to playing music, his passion. Whether he plays at home or away, his mother is always present at the performances; she is his best supporter. He is sorry about his social withdrawal and says that he would like to go out again more often, also because friends are very supportive and invite him out. As for the future, Malcom is positive. He says that as soon as he gets better, he will devote himself even more passionately to music. His dreams are to meet famous maestros, to become a composer, and to have a family. He tells the therapist that among the students of the conservatory there is a girl who plays the flute in whom he is particularly interested and whom he would like to invite out, if he only felt more self-confident, but he is positive and eager to succeed.

Malcom improves. He is better psychologically and reports a remission of the abdominal symptoms. The therapist regularly receives phone calls from Patricia, who enquires about her son's situation. Each time, the therapist kindly blocks these incursions.

After few months of continuous and gradual improvement, Malcom falls back into his negative thoughts and suffers from disabling abdominal pain again. The mother is at his side, and they spend another whole day in the emergency room.

The therapist reflects on the therapeutic process developed so far, and following the principle of interdependence, observes that she cannot help Malcom if, at the same time, she does not take account of the changes that Malcom's autonomy evokes in those to whom he is related. If Malcom were better, how would the relationship between him and his mother change? Patricia wants good for her son, but, on a deeper and more unconscious level, she might perceive Malcom's leaving home as threatening. From this perspective, Malcom's symptoms (which activate his mother), become protective of the stability of their relationship. From what has emerged during therapy, Malcom is ready to grow up and face the future, but his worsening at this moment may signal that he is not willing to do so at the expense of someone else's suffering, in particular that of his mother, for whom Malcom's autonomy might be felt as a loss.

The therapist communicates these thoughts to Malcom and asks his opinion about inviting his parents to the next session; he agrees and comments that his mother will be very happy to come, whereas he imagines that his father will be more reluctant. The parents accept the invitation. Their attitudes reflect what Malcom had predicted: mother is like a river in flood, whereas the father maintains an aloof position. The therapist shares with the parents the positive development achieved by their son, emphasizing that, given his many resources, he will certainly be able to overcome the difficult but significant moment he is going through. She also explains that she called them in because she is interested in what they think about it and how they see their and their son's future. Then, she asks Randal, the father, how he sees the relationship between Patricia and his son; Randal says, without thinking too much, that they are very close and that his wife treats him like a small child, while in his opinion, the son should be encouraged to step outside the family. Patricia, while crying, explains what becoming a mother meant for her and how much she feels connected to her son. Randal acknowledges that he has not been very present, that he devotes a lot of his time to work, and that he has delegated his parental role to his wife, especially in recent years. Noting Randal's tone of veiled regret, the therapist asks him if he would like to be more present, to be closer to his wife in a moment like this, in which Malcom is growing up and sooner or later will undertake his own way. At first, Randal seems thoughtful. Then, he describes projects that he would like to share with his wife. At the end of the session, the therapist underlines how each of them has needs and desires: Malcom has the desire to grow and accomplish his career as a musician; Patricia has the need to not feel lonely; Randal has the need to feel well-liked. The time has come for their needs and desires to be met.

The encounter ends with intense emotions and everyone's relief. The therapist, while declaring herself available for any future encounter, does not consider it necessary to plan others with the parents; she resumes individual sessions with Malcom to continue the path towards his autonomy, after having taken charge of the needs that Malcom's own autonomy produced for the significant people to whom he is attached.

When help entails taking account of the client's need not to be helped

Sometimes mutual loyalties in families are so strong that they override the need to pursue personal well-being. These are cases in which all members of the group are suffering for some reason. Unlike situations in which there is one or more person consensually designated as needing help and the others as those helping, there are circumstances in which all members of the network of significant relationships find themselves for some reason in the position of helping and being helped simultaneously, with the risk of activating a dynamic that can lead to a stalemate: each person feels the duty to protect the others from their own pain so as not to burden the already difficult situation the others are experiencing; each one takes on the suffering of the other, with the paradoxical result that everyone denies their own pain, which prevents the other from activating help. This is the case for families who experience the early death of a child or of a parent while still parenting children in their developmental years. Each person is faced with the sense of emptiness that follows the loss of their loved one, but also the pain of witnessing the condition of suffering in which other survivors find themselves, and therefore the desire to alleviate that suffering. Situations marked by such a coexistence of conflicting needs and feelings can also be found whenever a family must deal with multiple critical events; for example, while one faces an illness, another loses the job.

The therapist called upon to intervene in these cases is often asked by someone to take care of someone else, who is nevertheless more concerned about the former. Adopting the triadic perspective suggested in this chapter, the situation is stalled from the start. In fact, the interplay of mutual protectiveness prevents the negotiation of the very goal of therapy. The desire of one individual to take care of his /her problems is experienced as disinterest in the pain of the other who, however, avoids being the object of attention and care, commissioning the therapist to help the relative instead. It is a stalemate in which the activation of a positive co-evolutionary process for all members of the system implies that the therapist takes on the need of each one to withdraw from help, as in the following case.

Norman, 55 years old, contacted a therapist asking for the possibility of evaluating the beginning of a program for his mother Pauline, 76 years old, who was recently diagnosed with a neurodegenerative disease. During the phone call, Norman emphasized that the family has been experiencing a period of great stress for about 1 year, and he feared that the situation could aggravate his mother's precarious health conditions. An initial appointment is scheduled with the presence of both mother and son.

Norman and Pauline live in 2 neighbouring apartments, which are next to each other. About 10 years ago, Pauline was widowed, and when her son got married, he and his wife moved to an apartment next to Pauline. Since then, Norman has been discreetly taking care of his mother's well-being. Their well-established balance was shattered about a year ago when Norman's wife, Melissa, died suddenly in a car accident. The event devastated Norman, who was deeply in love with his wife, as well as Pauline, who was fond of her daughter-in-law, whom she considered a daughter. To make matters worse, Melissa's parents have started a legal battle against Norman to have access to all their daughter's assets. To avoid the pain of being involved in a never-ending fight, Norman has agreed to renounce the inheritance, but the legal proceedings are still in progress. Norman says that the thing that makes him suffer the most in this situation is his mother's suffering, whereas for himself he feels confident that he will be able to face the legal proceedings.

Pauline, on the other hand, fears that Norman's in-laws may take him to court, and the latter's reassurances are ineffective. Pauline is not worried about her own illness, which she minimizes by comparing it to other illnesses with which she has been living for years; Pauline is worried about Norman's loneliness. During the session, the son minimized his mother's concern, defined as a "typical mother's concern", claiming that he would not be the first or last person to live alone. Despite the initial request for therapy for Pauline alone, mother and son continued to come together for a few meetings, and it became increasingly clear to the therapist that the deep bond that unites them was preventing them from getting in touch with their own distress. Pauline is unable to do what would reassure her son, that is, to talk about the disorientation and fear that the diagnosis has caused her, nor to think of the future scenarios that the disease envisages – actions that would reassure her son – because she feels she must help Norman to overcome the loss of his wife and to cope with her family's obstinacy. At the same time, Norman feels that he cannot express his fragility, nor can he get in touch with the pain resulting from his wife's loss and the attitude of the in-laws, or experience mourning – actions that would reassure his mother – because he wants to support his mother with respect to the fear deriving from her diagnosis and the progression of the disease. At this time, both would benefit from a therapeutic context in which to address these issues, but how can the therapist help them re-adjust their relationship so that time for themselves is not perceived as an abandonment of the other? How can the therapist help them make sure that the deep relationship that unites them can be a resource for reciprocal support instead of being a source of reciprocal painful worries?

Reading the situation with the model of co-evolution, it emerges that therapy is also stalled. Conducting joint meetings, in fact, reinforces the positions of mutual protection and leaves little room for the emergence of personal needs. At the same time, proposing separate therapeutic paths risks frightening them, since neither of them is ready to define themself as needing individual therapy: they accept being in therapy only for the sake of the other. To be able to help them experience their suffering, the therapist must take on the need that each of them feels to protect the other, by avoiding help. So, she decides to propose they come together for sessions, but enter the therapy room individually, one after the other. With Norman, the therapist explores the mother's point of view, helping him to see how the mother's peace of mind is linked to being able to think that the son can manage without her. Together, they reflect on ways in which he could reassure his mother by taking time for himself and showing her that he is not isolating himself. With Pauline, the meetings focus on Norman's experiences, and in the dialogue with the therapist, she can see how her son is concerned about his mother's future and the progression of the disease. They explore the social and interpersonal resources that Norman could lean on to take care of his mother's health-related needs. The therapist and Pauline then work on the possibility that she might agree to have someone help her in everyday life, to reassure her son that she, too, cares about her own health and listens to his advice.

As the meetings continue, together but separate, Pauline and Norman begin to make their first experiments in "mutual reassurance". Norman starts to go out with friends; Pauline agrees to have someone help her for a few hours a day. Both appear more relaxed towards each other. Gradually, the therapist notices a change: in the sessions, Pauline talks less about her son, whom she sees more engaged outside and less lonely; she begins instead to address her feelings of fear about illness and death. Norman, who sees his mother entrusted to a network and willing to be helped, begins to face the frozen grief and emotions related to the loss of his wife. Being able to take care, separately, of each other's feelings, which were recursively directed toward themselves, is what allowed this situation to unblock. Pauline and Norman would not have been able to devote time to their own fragilities if they had continued to think that by doing so, they were not taking care of the other. However, precisely by working in coherence with the principles of interdependence and co-evolution, each person's concern for the other's well-being became a resource rather than a constraint and allowed both to have access to their own experiences.

Acknowledging the context that we have discussed in this chapter is a competency based on the principle of co-evolution and allows therapists to have a vision about the meaning that, for the processes of relational interdependence, their intervention can take in the context of the client's life. In the next chapter, we will reflect instead about the positioning of the therapist with respect to the extended context of therapy itself.

References

Bateson, G. (ed.) [1961], *Percival's narrative*, Palo Alto, Stanford University Press.

Bateson, G. [1972], *Steps to an ecology of mind*, New York, Chandler.

Bateson, G. [1975], *Some aspects of socialization by trance*, in Ethos, 3, pp. 143–155.

Bronfenbrenner, U. [1979], *The ecology of human development*, Cambridge MA, Harvard University Press.

Fruggeri, L. [1998], *Famiglie. Dinamiche interpersonali e processi psico-sociali*, Roma, Carocci.

Rober, P. [2017], *In therapy together*, London, Palgrave.

9 Constructing networks

The systemic nature of multi-professional interventions

The concepts of interdependence and co-evolution discussed in Chapter 8 can also be applied to cases that are involved with different agencies. When a network of professionals is involved in a case, clients and their families develop significant relationships with the professionals in charge of the treatment. In highly risky or multi-problematic situations, a "system of care" is activated. In these situations, what happens in the context of the relationship between one professional and the client reverberates on the client's significant systems, but also on the relationship between the client and the other professionals involved, then, circularly, on the relationship between the other professionals and the first one. In this sense, the boundaries of the therapist–client–significant others relationship should be expanded to include the interventions provided by the professional from the different agencies potentially involved. In such interdependent systems, each professional should become aware of her position as part of a therapeutic whole and act accordingly [Campbell and Draper 1985; Cecchin and Fruggeri 1986; Fruggeri and Matteini 1988; Fruggeri *et al.* 1991]. This competency helps therapists to analyze the complex network of relationships in which they as well as their clients participate, thereby allowing therapists to avoid the fragmentation, the interruption, or even the iatrogenic effect of their interventions.

Therapists aware of the implied different contexts can embrace a co-evolutionary approach that can guide them during interventions involving different agencies. More specifically, therapists embracing this perspective can be supported:

- To consider the impact of the treatment provided by all professionals involved in the case on the relationships between the client, the significant others in the clients' living context, and the professionals involved
- To organize the intervention considering not only what can be useful and transformative for clients and their relational systems, but also what can be useful and transformative for clients as part of a system of care with different professional roles involved.

DOI: 10.4324/9781003278092-14

In this sense, interdependence and coevolution become key systemic concepts also in complex interventions involving a network of agencies.

In Italy, where we work, mental health services for both adults and children and adolescents have many different components that serve different needs. Adult psychiatric agencies provide: outpatient service, home-based treatments, and consultancy; definition and implementation of rehabilitation and social care programmes; intervention in emergency situations; prescription, verification, and evaluation of admissions to the psychiatric unit; and psychological and pharmacological therapies. Mental health centres are also in contact with residential and semi-residential homes, as well as hospital wards for acute psychiatric treatments. Children and adolescents can rely on child psychiatry services, which have the mandate for: prevention, diagnosis, treatment, and rehabilitation of neurological, neuropsychological, psychological, and psychiatric problems. Both adult and child mental health services are supported by various private consultants who can be contacted directly by clients, or clients can be referred to them for the provision of specific therapeutic treatments.

Within this scenario, complex clinical cases – namely those requiring different levels of interventions, such as social care, drugs, and psychotherapy – should be based on the coordination of different professionals in charge of delivering the different treatments. Professionals should be able to analyze the complexity deriving from the contribution of each of them and acknowledge how every professional can be a resource for the client. The Open Dialogue approach builds upon this idea. Open dialogue is a community-based approach in which all the resources identified in the clients' context are mobilized for the planning and delivery of the intervention (see Box 9.1).

Box 9.1　Open Dialogue as a community approach by Jimmy Ciliberto

At the beginning of the 1990s, in the international journals of psychiatry and psychotherapy, practitioners started talking about Open Dialogue to describe a modality, developed in 1984 in Finland for taking care of critical psychiatric situations. Jaakko Seikkula and colleagues, influenced by the systemic approach to family therapy, by the Need Adapted Treatment and by Bakhtin's reflection on polyphony and dialogue [1984], decided to radically change the entire organization of the psychiatric services. The new organization, which still exists today [Seikkula *et al.* 2003], is an example of community psychiatry based on the respect of 7 principles:

1　Immediate help: patients are taken care of as soon as possible, accepting the definition of crisis that the client gives, whatever it is; the crisis is not feared, but valued and considered as a generative moment, in which the patient has the opportunity to express those contents that, usually, remain unheard.

2   Social network perspective: individuals are not considered as monads detached from the influences of the contexts; consequently, all the people who are significant to patients are invited to facilitate the therapeutic process.

3   Flexibility and mobility: the meetings can vary with respect to the number of voices present; the place where they take place is also chosen from time to time together with patients and their families. The sufferings of patients have unique characteristics and needs and, consequently, require flexible responses.

4   Responsibility of the team

5   Psychological continuity: professionals always guarantee a first meeting, regardless of the type of concern, and make decisions on the treatment always and only in the presence of the patients. It is essential to entrust the case to a team of 2 or 3 professionals, who will become the reference for one patient and his/her network, also in the face of a new crisis. These 2 aspects become effective antidotes against the extreme fragmentation of services and the increasing precariousness of professionals, which often determine a reduced ability to tune in and respond to the needs of the community.

6   Tolerance of uncertainty and

7   Dialogism: the first 5 principles build a sort of network, sufficiently secure, to help professionals and patients tolerate uncertainty, that is, the ability to listen and take time to co-construct the most suitable healing process for that system. During the meeting, it becomes essential to create the conditions to foster vertical and horizontal polyphony, that is, the ability to give space to the different voices that dwell within each of us, and then put them in dialogue with the different voices that inhabit the people who participate in the meeting.

Managing complex cases with different professionals involved requires having a strong conceptual framework that can account for the interdependence of professionals' interventions. In fact, planning meetings to exchange information among the professionals of the agencies involved is not enough: professionals should reflect on how their intervention connects with that of other professionals and acknowledge and value the differences of all actors involved. In other words, professionals should become aware of being part of an interdependent system and work within that framework, adopting a co-evolutionary perspective. However, given this complexity, the risk of opting for pragmatic solutions is just around the corner. For instance, one professional part of the network might take on the role of the "manager" to control the work of the other professionals involved. This could be seen as an attempt to build a network; instead, it is a pragmatic solution to manage complexity, which reduces it by controlling what the others do. The implication of this solution is the opposite of what should be aimed for when working in a network of agencies; therefore, the risk is causing reciprocal damage. The case illustrated below exemplifies this risk.

Alice is a 15-year-old girl hospitalized in a rehabilitation facility after a suicide attempt, which occurred after repeated episodes of severe self-injury. The psychiatrist in charge of the rehabilitation plan suggests the parents undertake family therapy. Alice's mother contacts a private family therapist in response to the advice given by the medical team in charge of Alice's case, since she trusts them. After obtaining the clients' consent, the therapist contacts Dr. Smith – the psychiatrist – to explore the reasons that prompted him to suggest family therapy. Dr. Smith reports that, according to him, Alice's problems relate to an unstable family scenario, in which she cannot find adequate support for her development. Accordingly, he thinks that family therapy could help the parents coordinate their parenting better. Alice's family includes her mother, Elisabeth, and her father Stephen: they have been divorced for 7 years. Alice lives with her mother. Elisabeth has had a new partner, Marc, for 5 years; Marc does not live with Elisabeth and Alice, but he often stays overnight on weekends. Stephen is unemployed and lives in a nearby town. After the divorce, he has had only occasional contact with Alice because of severe depression that has affected him since he lost his job. Recently, he has expressed interest in having more contact with his daughter.

For the first session, the therapist invites Alice's biological family. Since the very first exchanges, the therapist notes that the mother and father can hardly coordinate as parents. The father considers Alice's problems to be typical of adolescence, so not particularly worrying; in his view, time and good will would easily solve the problems. The mother, who appears to be a cold-looking woman, acknowledges her daughter's problems, but she responds with anger when Alice refuses to talk; this makes Alice even more distant from her mother, who in turn feels helpless. Elizabeth reports that she has always felt alone in parenting her daughter, and such a feeling has lately intensified since Stephen does not want to be involved in Alice's treatment because he "does not believe in psychology". After some sessions with Alice, Elisabeth, and Stephen, and building upon Dr. Smith's hypothesis, the therapist decides to invite Elisabeth and Marc for a session to explore Marc's role in Alice's up-bringing. Marc appears fond of Alice and empathetic with her problems. However, he says he has always been very cautious with being involved in Alice's issues since in the past Stephen accused him of interfering with his family; therefore, he fears that being more involved would cause further confusion to Alice. The therapist decided to start psychotherapy with Elisabeth, Marc, and Alice and – liaising with the professionals of the rehabilitation facility – decided to work on how Alice's symptoms might link to lack of security with respect to the new couple, who might not have looked solid enough in Alice's eyes. The sessions focus on helping Elizabeth and Marc to strengthen their couple relationship as well as the parenting functions within a family context of multiple households that involve stepparenting[1].

Psychotherapy continues for a couple of months with some improvements on Alice's part: she was discharged from the rehab centre and went back to school. At this point in time, Alice is in treatment with a child psychiatrist and a psychologist and receives support from educators of the after-school service. Each professional continues to work individually and has no chance to meet and talk to one another. Alice's health has improved, self-injury behaviours disappeared; however, she continues to show binge-eating behaviours. The child psychiatrist and the psychologist interpret Alice's symptom as an attempt to attract her biological father's attention. Also, believing that family therapy was not going anywhere, the child psychiatrist and the psychologist invited Elisabeth to tell the family therapist that Marc should no longer be involved in the sessions and instead Stephen should be invited. What was happening?

The complexity of Alice's case required the collaboration of professionals from different agencies; however, no contact had occurred, and no plans had been discussed. Professionals worked in parallel for a while, but with the emergence of Alice's new symptom, discrepancies emerged among the professionals. The child psychiatrist took the role of the "manager" – something that had not been negotiated and that was not part of any protocol – and tried to control Alice's therapeutic plan. However, in so doing she unwittingly disempowered the family therapy treatment that was going well. The family therapist, on her part, felt she had to safeguard her work with Alice's family, but in so doing, she was disqualifying the psychiatrist's professional role. In the meantime, Alice's symptom was getting worse. In other words, by working independently and with no coordination, even if with the same aim of offering support to Alice, professionals were reproducing the same pattern that Alice was experiencing in her family context: adults not being able to provide care and protection to her. Prompted by the increasing severity of Alice's symptom, the family therapist proposed to set up a meeting.

Meetings among professionals involved in a clinical case are important occasions in which to make sense of the different interventions, draw connections among them, and re-design the therapeutic plan that is at the same time multi-dimensional and unitary. In fact, during the meeting, the professionals agree that Alice should explore her emotional problems in individual therapy so that family therapy could continue to focus on improving the communication among the multiple households of Alice's family. The possibility of discussing the case in a meeting has allowed all professionals to see that the fragmentation of their interventions was amplifying Alice's problem instead of reducing it. Thanks to this meeting, the professionals were able to re-organize their interventions and set the basis for the development of an integrated and collaborative plan. The child psychiatrist, who at that point had become aware of the goal of family therapy, decided to align with the family therapist in keeping the biological father, Stephen, involved since he trusted the pharmacological therapy prescribed by the child psychiatrist, whereas the family therapist would continue to work with Alice, Elisabeth and Marc. Individual therapy allowed Alice to talk about the pain of her father's absence; family therapy sessions strengthened Alice's family context and prepared it to sustain Alice's vulnerabilities. Also, Alice could progressively acquire more autonomy and attend the after-school service where, with the support of educators, she could improve her relational skills for interacting with peers.

The illustration of this case shows that activating multiple interventions for a complex case is not enough for the positive outcome of the treatment. Alice could rely on several professionals who, guided by good intentions, wanted to help her, but this was not enough since neither a network nor a system of care was developed. In other words, all professionals involved worked within the premise that each professional was working independently on different therapeutic plans, thereby contributing to the fragmentation of the intervention. Yet, the idea of a "manager" deciding for all to avoid the fragmentation of interventions did not produce better results. Building a network of multiple professionals implies taking a complex perspective that acknowledges how therapeutic efficacy emerges from the relationship with the others. In fact, when finally meeting and talking to each other, all the single components of the therapeutic system began to think of themselves as part of a project to be constructed together through the identification of the connections among all the components.

Professionals' coordination in a therapeutic project

In multi-professional networks, therapeutic interventions should be developed by looking not at individual therapeutic objectives, but at a shared therapeutic plan. In an ecological perspective the questions that guide therapeutic interventions are not only "What meaning can this intervention have in the life of that client?" but also, "How does my intervention connect with that of my colleagues and impact on the life of that client?". Coordination within a therapeutic plan that consists of many elements, allows one to include the multiple and often conflicting needs of the clients and the people who belong to their relational networks. In the perspective of interdependence between different interventions, the roles of the various agencies involved in a case cannot be considered as limited to their ascribed functions or to a predefined organization. They should rather be flexible and adjust to the specific histories of clients and to the global therapeutic plan. This does not mean that the different therapeutic entities involved in a case should abandon their role. For instance, the family therapist will work with the whole family, the psychiatrist will prescribe drugs, educators will support socialization, the psychologist's intervention will target the client's individual needs, nurses of residential facilities will oversee the organization of clients' everyday activities during hospitalization, etc. It is rather a matter of identifying a framework in which the peculiarity of each service is defined with respect to that of the others. This implies that the different parts of the therapeutic system work as a team at the different stages of the intervention, namely: 1) analysis and formulation of a hypothesis concerning the case; 2) identification of the different needs; 3) identification of the meanings that each intervention takes with respect to the others for the clients; and 4) definition of the professionals involved in the case as a complex yet unified system of care that responds to clients' needs. Albert's case exemplifies this approach.

Albert, 18 years old, was admitted to an emergency service after he attempted suicide; shortly afterwards, he was transferred to a psychiatric ward. During the hospitalization, the psychologist of the hospital met Albert and his parents, Vincent and Ruby, who appeared reticent and were opposed to the psychologist's suggestion of transferring Albert to a residential facility. The parents wanted Albert to continue to attend school, which was the most important thing for them. Albert was evasive about school, which he had stopped attending before the suicide attempt. During the session with the psychologist, he was collaborative and provided useful information about his family, which allowed the therapist to develop a therapeutic plan. Albert's family had moved recently from another region where Vincent was born because Ruby had never been happy there and needed to look after her mother. Vincent managed to transfer his business, and they moved into an apartment near Ruby's mother. While talking about her mother, Ruby burst into tears: her mother had died a year earlier of heart disease, which was diagnosed too late. Ruby felt guilty; she accused herself of not having realized in time the severity of her mother's illness. The psychologist asked Albert if he was close to his grandmother and if he had suffered at her loss. Albert responded that he was very close to his grandmother but that they could only talk of his mother's pain. The psychologist commented as follows: "Albert, it must have been very difficult for you not being allowed to grieve since it was mum who needed support for her bereavement". Albert stared at the psychologist, and at the end of the session, he stated that he accepted going to the residential facility. The parents insisted that they would agree if he promised to go back to school. Albert did not answer. Moreover, during the interview, the parents mentioned that they felt blamed but that they had always acted for Albert's sake.

The transfer from the psychiatric ward to the residential facility required a meeting with the team of the professionals in charge of the case to discuss a therapeutic plan, namely the psychiatrist of the residential facility, the psychiatrist of the inpatient unit, the psychologist of the family therapy service, and the psychiatrist of the community mental health service. The professionals reflected on four points:

1   The information collected during the family interview indicated that the parents could not contain Albert's anxiety, and Albert was unable to control his own anxiety.

2   From Albert's feedback during the family interview, he felt "seen" in his emotional states by the psychologist, but the goal was to help his parents to "see" him.
3   Albert's ambivalence about going to school needed to be explored further: this issue seemed to activate his parents as if for Albert the school non-attendance was a way of attracting his parents' attention.
4   The parents looked defensive, felt judged, and did not seem willing to cooperate.

The professionals reflected on the fact that Albert's needs and his parents' needs were in conflict. Albert tried to highlight his emotional problems and to be supported for his anxieties; the parents felt this was a criticism to their parenting, and they defended themselves by shifting their concern to the school, which was a critical issue for Albert. It was clear that Albert's family, like any system that is based on distance, was dealing with a great level of suffering. In this sense, ambivalence and dysfunctional dynamics had to be replaced by reciprocal care and the creation of a context that could allow the free expression of individual needs. Building upon these considerations, the professionals decided that the treatment plan had to be twofold: supporting Albert's autonomy while in the rehab centre and working with the family to mobilize the resources that could support Albert in his recovery process. The psychiatrist of the community service guaranteed that the family would continue to receive support after Albert's discharge from the residential centre.

However, the problem of how to involve everyone in the project had to be addressed. Albert had already expressed his agreement to adhere to the program, but his parents appeared reluctant to engage; they felt judged and tended to be defensive. In these situations of different or conflicting needs, service networks and multi-professional teams are particularly useful since every service and role can respond to different needs, which are nevertheless interconnected by the professional collaborative work. With this in mind, the professionals decided that the psychiatrist of the rehab centre who was working on Albert's personal autonomy with socializing activities, group therapy, and psychopharmacological treatment, would keep the parents regularly informed through weekly meetings to update them on Albert's progresses and ask for their collaboration. In parallel, the family therapist would meet the parents and Albert to learn more about the problematic relational aspects that emerged in the first session. The two areas of intervention tackled interwoven triadic contexts that had complementary needs: in the context of the residential centre the psychiatrist and the parents coordinated to help Albert with gaining more autonomy, thereby connecting the personal development of Albert with the construction of better parental capacity and acknowledgement. In the family therapy sessions, the therapist favoured dialogue between Albert and his parents to explore what prevented them from mutual care and a sense of belonging, thereby supporting Albert's need to redefine family relationships. The professionals agreed to keep in touch to monitor and coordinate the development of the different interventions.

The acknowledgement of parents as interlocutors of Albert's therapeutic plan put them in a secure position that enabled their engagement in family therapy sessions. Similarly, the participation in family therapy sessions and the focus on family dynamics respected and valued Albert's point of view about the expression of his feelings towards his parents. The coordination of the interventions in such a manner started to give positive outcomes. Albert went back to school with the collaboration of his mother, who every morning called him on the phone to get him up to go to school. The residential centre psychiatrist's weekly sessions with the parents also continued with the aim of informing them about the rehab programme and ensuring their cooperation in that respect. Family therapy sessions favoured the development of new ways of communicating about the emotions between Albert and his parents and between the two partners. Focussing therapeutic conversations on other issues, the school was no longer at the centre of negotiating the definition of the relationship between Albert and his parents. Going back to school became an important activity for Albert's development through the support and collaboration of the team of the rehab centre team and of his parents. These initial positive changes opened a space for other issues relevant to the family to be discussed.

The family went through a very difficult period before deciding to leave the region where the parents had lived and got married. Moving to another region of the country allowed them to feel better, but they did not take the time to elaborate all the suffering they went through. Family therapy sessions created a space for progressively exploring that experience. When Ruby and Vincent got married, they moved to an apartment in the same building where Vincent's parents lived. After Albert's birth, the relationship between Ruby and her mother-in-law deteriorated. Ruby felt judged and controlled as if she was not a good mother. Ruby shared her discomfort with Vincent, asking him to take action and talk to his mother and tell her to stop controlling. Vincent sometimes told Ruby that his mother was not controlling and it probably was just Ruby's impression; some other times, he told her not to care about what his mother did or said. With the help of the therapist, it was possible for Ruby, Vincent, and Albert to talk about this delicate phase of their family's life, thereby transforming the conversations on these issues into an occasion for reconnecting the three of them. Vincent said he was sorry for not having understood Ruby's suffering; Albert explained he felt caught in the middle of the conflict between mother and father, when Ruby was asking Vincent to take a stand against his family. The family therapy sessions and the program of the rehab centre were helping them to untie relational and subjective knots. Things were progressing positively when close to discharge from the residential centre, Albert expressed his doubt to the psychologist: "I'm afraid that when I get home, everything will go back as before!". The professionals consulted and decided that it was time to move to a new phase: his parents had to reassure Albert that there was no risk of going back to where things were before. While Albert was continuing his rehabilitation program, it was decided that family therapy sessions would be attended by the parents only so that they could negotiate a new partnership agreement. Albert is now back home, and he behaves to everyone's satisfaction. He has undertaken an individual psychotherapy that can support him with the transition to adulthood.

Albert's case illustrates how by developing professional networks according to an ecological and social constructionist perspective, professionals can include and accommodate different needs without considering them as mutually exclusive or opposed. Through the activation of a multifaceted dynamic that includes the different services and the clients, it is possible to diversify the contexts of the intervention so that, for example, the need for autonomy can coexist with belonging; the needs of belonging, care, and protection can coexist with autonomy and individual growth; and emotions can coexist with rational reflection. The ability to keep these different parts together is one of the resources of the network. The multiplicity of contexts, if coordinated, can become therapeutic tools that allow all actors involved (clients and professionals) to experience that even irreconcilable aspects or needs can coexist (see Chapter 6). Complex thinking as a tool at the service of the network is the premise for the construction of generative contexts within which new stories and new solutions become possible.

Fostering information circularity

The coordination of multi-professional interventions requires moving from a dualistic "true vs. false" perspective to a circular one in which different and apparently contrasting events, emotions, and positions are recursively connected. The transition from one perspective to the other is fostered by the coordination of the different agencies involved but also by the ability to activate an exchange of information in which different observations on behalf of different professionals are considered as generative of complex thinking. The case described below illustrates these processes.

Christine is 15 years old; her parents, Lisa and Luke, separated 5 years ago, but their relationship is still conflictual. After the divorce, it was agreed that Christine would spend some days of the week at her mother's house and the other days at her father's house. Both parents were committed to an equitable division of their daughter's care. However, after a while some problems emerged.

When the mother started a new relationship and her new partner moved in, Christine wanted to spend more time with her father, both during the week and on the weekends. Also, she started to show problematic behaviours, such as: refusing to go to school, self-injuring by making cuts on her arms, and threatening suicide. She was referred to the local child psychiatry service that diagnosed her with an "emotionally unstable personality disorder". Christine was sent to a residential facility, where she was treated individually. After entering this service, the teenager stopped self-harming and seemed well-adjusted: she went to school, did her homework, and participated in group activities with her peers; however, she refused to see her parents during the time allocated for visits. The psychotherapist who had Christine under treatment felt stuck, since the teenager was oppositional and refused to explain the reason for not wishing to meet her parents. The psychotherapist's perspective did not match the observations of the educators of the residential facility, who considered Christine to be a cooperative and quiet girl. Meanwhile, the relationship between the parents was getting more hostile: according to the mother, her daughter's problems were linked to the conflictual dynamics of the parents, for which she blamed the father. The father, instead, explained Christine's problems as deriving from the mother's manipulations and, in his words, "parental alienation" behaviours.

Professionals faced contrasting scenarios: in one context, Christine appeared functional and happy; in another context, she was described as dysfunctional and suffering. Consequently, the psychotherapist felt caught in an impasse, while the educators were happy with the teenager's improvements. As for the parents, they "used" Christine's suffering to foster their conflictual relationship while looking for lineal explanations that would attribute responsibility to one person or to the other. While looking for "the truth", all actors were stuck.

Alongside this, the Court prescribed an assessment of Lisa's and Luke's parenting capacity; this introduced new difficulties into a system already characterized by oppositions. For this purpose, interviews were conducted with the parents separately to investigate their perception of the family system, rules, and boundaries. In addition, the psychologist in charge of the assessment asked to analyze the interactions between Christine and her parents all together. For this analysis, the Triadic Interaction Analytical Procedures (TIAP) [Venturelli et al. 2016; Venturelli et al. 2022] was used. The professionals thought that this was impossible to happen given Christine's refusal to meet her parents. Surprisingly, Christine agreed to see her parents when she realized that both were attending the session for the TIAP administration. This provided an important piece of information: what had been considered as Christine's refusal to see her parents, emerged as the refusal to see them separately. Christine and her parents met after several months of absence; however, the emotional climate was good among the 3 of them. They played together as indicated by the chosen procedure; they were engaged and collaborative. From analysis of the triadic interactions, it emerged that Christine and her parents worked well when the parents interacted with the daughter separately although in each other's presence. While daughter and father were playing, Lisa remained peripheral, and Christine and Luke looked highly connected without worrying too much about keeping the mother out of the interaction. Likewise, the interaction between mother and daughter was characterized by positive emotion and involvement, while Luke kept the position of a non-intrusive observer. The parents did not interfere with one another when playing with their daughter separately, thereby showing an absence of loyalty conflicts that would have prevented Christine from relating with her parents. Yet, since Christine agreed to see her parents when they were both present and given that the subsystems mother–daughter and father–daughter could function well separately but co-present, the professional thought that Christine needed to control what the other parent was doing while she was interacting with the one. This analysis was confirmed when family members were asked to play all together: the parents did not look at each other, they were not attentive to reciprocal and non-reciprocal signals, and they did not speak to each other directly. Christine, on her part, was active, attentive to everyone's needs, and directed the play, as if she had to make sure that there was no risk of conflict.

The analysis of triadic family interactions allowed the therapists to identify the characteristics of functional and dysfunctional family dynamics: Christine's symptoms and psychological problems could be seen as a way for her to communicate to her parents that she could no longer bear to regulate the tension between them. The placement in a residential facility became a sort of neutral space in which she could "rest" from the role of regulator of parental conflict. However, the placement did not allow her to solve the problematic relational dynamics in the family. This possible explanation for Christine's problem was also consistent with the fact that when in the residential structure, she was not manifesting the provocative behaviours that alarmed her parents and the professionals. This new information allowed for focussing on the function of the intervention of each service involved in the case.

The parenting assessment process became an opportunity to develop a common therapeutic plan that could involve different services and professionals and make sense of everyone's intervention. In a team meeting, which involved the social worker, the educators, Christine's psychologist, and the psychotherapist in charge of assessing parenting skills, it was decided that the latter would give to the Court and to the family the following messages: Christine will stay in the residential facility to continue to improve her relationship with her family by being distant from their conflict; she will resume individual psychotherapy with the therapeutic goal to work on her role and responsibilities within the family and with respect to her development; Lisa and Luke will be offered to have support in working on their conflictual relationship and to relieve Christine of the dysfunctional role of regulating their conflicts.

Christine's case can help professionals see that in different therapeutic contexts, people behave in different ways; in this sense, even contrasting behaviours should not be considered as opposed, but instead should be seen as the expression of a complex situation. From clients' perspective, professionals are not seen as separate; rather they are considered as active parts of a whole that creates different meanings and allows the expression of different parts of the Self [O'Sullivan 2021]. In other words, there is not "one, single" Christine. In different contexts, she can have different feelings and show different behaviours; professionals should be able to show Christine that differences can be connected.

Furthermore, the possibility of seeing that different contexts activate different parts of the self has a crucial role in building effective therapeutic networks. First, the information deriving from observation of clients' behaviour in one context also provides information on what should be done in other areas of intervention. In Christine's case, the information derived from the application of the TIAP during the parenting assessment process shed light on the meaning of Christine's behaviour in the residential care *and* in the individual therapy sessions. Furthermore, considering that every context offers the possibility of expressing different parts of the self implies considering that all the interventions activated (psychotherapeutic, pharmacological, educational, etc.) have the potential to trigger a positive process of change. However, this is linked to the ability of the involved professionals to analyze the meanings of the different interventions within the symbolic and relational context of the client. In this sense, supporting the circularity of information means working in connection with all professionals involved in the case to create a meaning-making process in which every part of the system contributes to co-construct.

The notion of "acknowledging the context", applied to the construction and the maintenance of multi-professional networks, highlights the fact that psychotherapy is not solely a process that takes place between a therapist and one or more clients; rather, it can be extended to include other professionals and other services, thereby emerging as an eco-system. The next chapter will show how while acknowledging the context, therapists also need to widen their gaze to how social and cultural contexts redefine individual and interpersonal relationships.

Note

1 Supporting stepfamilies implies: 1) strengthening the new couple bond, 2) creating a good relationship between stepparent and stepchildren, and 3) creating an alliance among the adults for the exercise of parenting (biological parents and new partners) [Visher, Visher and Parsley 2003].

References

Bachtin, M. [1984], *Problems of dostoevsky' poetics*, Minneapolis, University of Minnesota Press.

Cecchin, G. and Fruggeri, L. [1986], *Consultation with mental health systems teams in Italy*. In L. Wynne, S. Mcdaniel, and T. Weber (eds.) *The family therapist as systems consultant*, New York, The Guilford Press, pp. 103–114.

Campbell, D. and Draper, R. [eds] [1985], *Applications of systemic family therapy: the Milan Method*, London, Grune and Strutton.

Fruggeri, L. and Matteini, M. [1988], *Larger systems? Beyond a dualistic approach to the process of change*, The Irish Journal of Psychology, 9, 1, pp. 173–182.

Fruggeri, L., Telfener, U., Castellucci, A., Marzari, M. and Matteini, M. [1991], *New systemic ideas from the italian mental health movement*, London, Karnac Books.

O'Sullivan, B. [2021] *Working with a metaphor: creating relationship with self as a community of selves*, Dublin, Orpen Press.

Seikkula, J., Alakare, B., Aaltonen, J., Holma, J., Rasinkangas, A. and Lehtinen, V. (2003). *Open dialogue approach: treatment principles and preliminary results of a two-year follow-up on first episode schizophrenia.* Ethical Human Sciences and Services, 5, 3, pp. 163–182.

Venturelli, E., Cabrini, E., Fruggeri, L. and Cigala, A. [2016], *The study of triadic family interactions: the proposal of an observational procedure*, in Integrative Psychological Behavioral Science, 50, 4, pp. 655–683.

Venturelli, E., Fruggeri, L. and Cigala, A. [2022], *Valutazione del funzionamento familiare. La prospettiva triadica della procedura TIAP*, Milano, Raffaello Cortina.

Visher, E.B., Visher, J.S. and Pasley, K. [2003], *Remarriage families and stepparenting*, in F. Walsh (ed.), *Normal family processes (3rd edition)*, New York, The Guilford Press, pp. 153–175.

10 The multi-process analysis

In the previous chapters, we have illustrated how psychotherapy takes place in the interweaving of meanings and interactions that characterize the relationship between client and therapist, the clients, relationships with their own system of belonging, and with other eventual professionals involved.

However, the context of interpersonal relationships is not the only one impacting the trajectory of personal development. Individuals and their systems grow within a web of processes that connect personal features to inter-personal aspects, and both to socio-economic-political-institutional structures. Factors such as social and cultural affiliations, power relations, material conditions of existence, dominant ideologies, socio-economic processes, norms, and values that validate and maintain the social order, are not a background to the development of individual paths; they are factors that, intertwining with personal characteristics and with the quality of interpersonal relationships, define the well-being of individuals and the functioning of the group to which they belong. From this point of view, acknowledging the context implies that a therapist adopts a multi-process approach, which involves considering the interdependence of individual, interpersonal, and social processes in defining the well-being or distress of individuals. Acknowledging the context, in this sense, means considering how the social dimension of people's existence can influence the development of discomfort, and how necessary it is to keep it in mind both in the process of hypothesizing and exploration of clients' stories, and in the implementation of the intervention. In this sense, " ... the inclusion of wider contextual factors, including political-historical power structures, will be seen to be an intrinsic part of what assures a therapist's responsible attention to all relevant issues which organize and influence the lives and the well-being of clients" [Jones 1993, p. 150].

The social dimension affecting people's lives can be understood in two different ways: as the web of social, economic, political, cultural, and institutional processes through which people live their individual and inter-personal experiences; or as the set of expectations, ideologies, stereotypes, prejudices, and social representations that contribute to regulate and structure the processes of the personal and inter-subjective sphere as well as the public and collective one.

DOI: 10.4324/9781003278092-15

Individual well-being and social status

One of the most significant and well-established findings of scholarly research in recent decades is the confirmation of the negative impact that economic problems have on the dynamics of families and on the development of their members [Conger, Conger and Martin 2010]. Empirical research has described the cascading process that connects family socioeconomic status, individuals' emotional reactions, relationships among members, and individual development. In poor families, economic shortcomings cause constant daily tension in parents with respect to their ability to provide expenses and needs (bills, rent, school fees, medical expenses, etc.) for the family; this tension translates into emotional distress for both partners, leading to increased fighting between them, couple dissatisfaction, and emotional distancing; fighting, dissatisfaction, and distancing, in turn, reverberate negatively on the quality of relationships between parents and children, increasing conflict and chaos in the family environment, thereby jeopardizing the well-being of the latter as well [Cui, Donnellan and Conger 2007; Nelson *et al.* 2009]. In other cases, other authors have found that daily economic pressure triggers depressive reactions in parents, reducing their perception of their own effectiveness and generating a sense of worthlessness, which has repercussions on the quality of care they provide for their children, who are therefore exposed to growing conditions characterized by widespread distress [Nievar and Luster 2006]. Equally interesting are clinical studies that have traced the relationship between depression, female gender, and socioeconomic conditions. Women's depressive symptoms may be a normal reaction to intolerable life circumstances such as isolation, poverty, inadequate housing, marginalization, and inability to provide for the needs of their children [Jones 1994].

All these contributions support the conclusions of the many authors who, already in the 1990s, denounced psychotherapeutic models based on a-historical and a-political premises, which interpret and treat psychological discomfort exclusively as the result of personal characteristics or relational dynamics. Ignoring the differences created by unequal power relations and disparities in the ability to access resources, leads psychotherapists to replicate and reinforce such differences through their interventions, as well as to perpetuate the oppression and discrimination that such differences entail [Walters 1990; McCarthy 1995; Pakman 1997]. The connection between powerlessness and psychological distress calls for therapeutic interventions that are geared towards making clients proactive in coping with the difficult circumstances in which they live [McCarthy 1994]. This may involve having conversations about these issues in the therapeutic context and offering clients information, reflections, and analyses that can enable them to act in order to bring about change, including social change. In these cases, therapeutic intervention aims to shift the origin of one's discomfort from oneself to the social context, that is, to produce awareness of the effect that this level has on personal psychological conditions. A psychotherapeutic intervention cannot in itself change social conditions; however, it can help generate awareness that can then be acted upon by clients in the social context [Afuape 2016].

Economic conditions are not the only factor that affects people's psychological and physical well-being. Research documented that racism has deep negative psychosocial and physical health consequences [Brondolo *et al.* 2008; Williams and Mohammed 2009]. Racism or ethnic discrimination can include acts such as social exclusion, workplace discrimination, stigmatization, physical threat, harassment, abuse, and personal violence. Racism may have deleterious effects, even when the target does not consciously perceive the maltreatment or attribute it to racism [Brondolo *et al.* 2009]. It is important for the psychotherapist to recognize how psychological distress of people belonging to a discriminated ethnic community can have its root in racism. Drawing on Liberation Psychology, Afuape and Kerry Oldham [2022, p. 25] suggest that in order to support emotional well-being of discriminated people it is essential to "explicitly name oppression and link it to emotional distress; connect to a social and collective history of how people have challenged oppression in the past that can be used today; draw on the resources, forms of resistance, creativity and resilience of oppressed people". As outlined by Chin *et al.* [2022], an antiracist and decolonizing practice is a collaborative practice in as much as it recognizes and acknowledges the ways clients have developed to resist the structural inequities connected to racism. Systemic practitioners can rely on methods and techniques that favour a stance of curiosity and dialogue (see Chapter 2) and can recognize the oppression that they face and draw on the resourceful resisting strategies that they develop.

In addition, extreme conditions such as those experienced in contexts of war or persecution produce in people a suffering whose meaning can only be found in a complex web of political, cultural, relational, and psychological experiences that therapists must recognize and legitimize (see Box 10.1). Doing therapy with asylum seekers, victims of collective violence, or survivors of ethnic persecution requires therapists to take a politically aware stance that allows them to construct with clients a dialogical space that explicitly acknowledges the political origin of the experiences of intentional de-humanization and de-culturation suffered by these people [Sironi 2007]. When working with individuals who have lived experiences of collective violence, psychotherapeutic competency must be integrated and enhanced by knowledge of the international political, historical, economic, and legal events that are at the source of the clients' suffering so that the therapist is able to interact with them and accompany them through their description of the violence, reconstruction and clarification of the political responsibility of the aggressors, and recognition of the resistance strategies implemented against the perpetrated violence, thus activating the process of recovery of their violated identity [Sironi 2007; Davolo and Fruggeri 2016].

Box 10.1   The specificity of trauma from collective violence

Trauma from collective violence is an intentional trauma, deliberately induced by someone, and therefore contains a political dimension that refers to the political objectives of the aggressor. Failure to take this into account risks generating authentic forms of reactive paranoia in patients, caused by situations of mistreatment attributable to inadequate theories, practices, or therapeutic devices [Sironi 2007].

The definition of Post-Traumatic Stress Disorder taken from the *Diagnostic and Statistical Manual of Mental Disorders* (DSM), used in the Western psychiatric classification, is inadequate with respect to the experience lived by these patients. According to the American Psychiatric Association [2002] the essential feature of post traumatic stress disorder is the development of typical symptoms that follow direct personal experience of an event that causes or may result in death or serious injury, or other threats to physical integrity. This definition, however, does not distinguish the fact that, in the case of collective violence, the traumatic event was deliberately induced with the intentional political goal of de-culturing people and destroying their personal, social, cultural, and human identity. In this sense, a psychotherapeutic intervention cannot ignore the fact that patients have undergone a process of de-humanization and de-culturation. A therapeutic intervention that descends integrally and directly from the classical theory of trauma, runs the risk of using procedures that, in the eyes of individuals who have been subjected to techniques of subjugation, may reproduce the initial conditions of the traumatizing situation (interrogations, torture) and the "state-citizen" relations typical of dictatorial or tyrannical political regimes.

For these reasons, it is necessary, in the specific case of the treatment of trauma from collective violence with applicants/holders of international protection, to build a dialogical space with the patient, which allows the explicit recognition in therapy of the political significance of the trauma [Sironi 2007; Davolo and Mancini 2017]. Such a stance is also ethical and is necessary for the deconstruction of the condition of subjugation and totalitarian influence as the first step towards the recovery of identity erased by intentional trauma [for an example of a therapy conducted according to these principles with a refugee victim of collective violence in the context of civil war in her country, see the case in Davolo and Fruggeri 2016, pp. 121–122].

Another example of collective violence is that perpetrated against black and brown people, highlighted recently by Black Lives Matter. Also in this case, psychotherapists recognize the political significance of the trauma, overtly take an ethical stance against racism, and voice their

> political opinions as a condition for helping people who have suffered
> the impact of intergenerational racism to "re-author the story of their
> lives to bring about healing" [Afuape *et al.* 2022, p. 8].

Personal psychological discomfort due to social circumstances can be found
in many other cases: exposure to systematic humiliation or marginalization in
the workplace; being the object of constant ethnic, religious, or sexual discrimination; or falling victim to a repeated and unpunished violation of human
rights. These are all cases that cannot be addressed without helping clients to
understand their personal experiences in the broader discourse of human and
civil rights. Therapists cannot replace those who have public responsibility for
enforcing these rights, but they can work with their clients so that they first
develop a self-respect that enables them to connect to a broader movement
capable of challenging those who have responsibility for implementing rights
[McDowell, Libal and Brown 2012].

In this sense, in therapies with people whose suffering derives from the lack of
respect for inalienable rights, from abuse of power, from racism, from poor
existential conditions, or from circumstances that annihilate their agency, it is
central: 1) to recognize that the responsibility for their discomfort lies outside
themselves and reconstruct the process that created the discomfort; 2) to
promote competence and resilience through dialogues that bring out the ways in
which they, even in suffering, have resisted the difficulties; and 3) to identify the
collective context within which they can take action, in order to feel legitimized
in their demand for recognition as rightful subjects [Todds and Wade 2003].

Social knowledge, interpersonal dynamics, and individual well-being

The study of the impact of discrimination, due to prejudices and stereotypes,
on individual development and on interpersonal psychological dynamics is
another field of investigation that confirms the need to adopt a multi-process
perspective in doing psychotherapy. Let us read the following case and then
reflect on it.

Isabel is 35 years old; she is a worker in a textile industry. She lives with her
parents and has 2 older sisters who are married with children. She consults a
psychotherapist because lately she has been afraid to go out; she feels very tense
and lives with a constant feeling of impending danger. She continues to work
regularly but has greatly reduced her social life.

The significant figures Isabel describes to the therapist are her parents, to
whom she is very close and with whom she has always lived in a small town in
a province of central Italy; her sisters, who, she claims, have been an important
point of reference for her and who have encouraged her to see a psychologist;
and 32-year-old Hannah, whom Isabel describes with some embarrassment as

her best friend. Hannah is married and has a 5-year-old daughter, Lynn. When encouraged by the therapist to talk more about Hannah, Isabel explains that they met at work and have developed an intense emotional relationship over the past year or so. Isabel has also become a familiar figure to Hannah's daughter, as the 2 women and the child sometimes share moments of leisure. Over the last year, their relationship has become more and more intense, and Hannah, whose relationship with her husband was already critical before she met Isabel, is thinking of separating. Hannah and Isabel are planning to live together in the future, with Lynn – subject to the divorce agreement.

Neither her parents nor her sisters know about this relationship and – Isabel points out – they will never have to find out. The parents are still in good shape, but they are getting older, and she doesn't want to worry them. Isabel says that she can't even imagine what her parents' reaction would be if they knew she is having a love affair with a woman. Isabel expresses her will to continue the relationship with Hannah and her desire to build a life together, but she feels very tense and anxious, and at this moment, she is not able to make any decision.

A month later, Isabel presents an aggravation of her symptoms: she reports panic attacks. Hannah has communicated to her husband her intention to divorce and has temporarily gone to live with her daughter at a friend's house in a nearby city, waiting to find an apartment where Isabel can join them. Hannah has started to attend LGBT+ support groups, and Isabel is annoyed. She reports confusion, indecision, and insecurity. She feels stuck; she is no longer sure she wants to continue the relationship with Hannah.

While Isabel is more and more undecided, Hannah makes progress in defining herself as gay and in planning her life openly as a couple with Isabel (she looks for an apartment for both, attends the gay community's activities, and has contacted same-sex families' associations for advice on same-sex parenting). Hannah's acceleration has had a paralyzing effect on Isabel, who, in fact, feels completely blocked with respect to her life with Hanna.

What holds Isabel back with respect to the life she envisioned together with Hannah? Should Isabel's doubts about her relationship with Hannah be treated as an expression of a weakening of their relationship or should they be understood within other contexts of meaning? Because of homophobic prejudices and of the subsequent discriminatory attitudes, psychotherapists working with the LGBT+ population should consider a plurality of factors that are at the same time intrapersonal, interpersonal, and social. In this sense, we can respond to the above questions at different levels.

Faced with the possibility of implementing a plan hitherto only hypothesized or fantasized about until that moment, perhaps Isabel felt an uncertainty linked to the definition of herself as gay. The emotional involvement with Hannah, which took place in a way that was as intense as it was unexpected, had perhaps not allowed a deeper reflection at the identity level. From this point of view, the doubt as to whether to continue the relationship with Hannah could hide Isabel's uncertainty regarding the definition of her sexual orientation and identity.

Alternatively, Hannah's request to "make a family" opened a theme that Isabel had not yet faced with respect to the process of autonomy from her parents. Who would take care of them from now on, just when they are beginning the most fragile phase of their lives? Perhaps Isabel feels a sense of gratitude towards them, a loyalty that she feels to be competing with the construction of her own couple or family life.

Or, furthermore, Isabel feels that the negative social judgement about same-sex relationships is insurmountable to face with her parents. Defining oneself as a gay and following one's feelings of love towards a person of the same sex can have heavy personal and relational consequences in an Italian provincial environment. From this point of view, Isabel's paralysis with respect to her own life choices can be traced back to the need to not make her parents suffer for what she is, the need to defend her parents from herself. This feeling does not derive from an unfinished identity process or from a difficulty in freeing herself from her family of origin, but from the negative prejudice socially shared towards LGB+ people. To discern the importance of the social level in this case, the question to ask is: how different would it be if Isabel planned to move in with a man instead of Hannah? In other words, how much does social judgement about homosexuality regulate Hannah's personal and relational decisions?

The three levels of individual, interpersonal, and social processes are interconnected; however, for therapeutic purposes, it is necessary to identify, case by case, which level gives meaning to the whole plot [Rigliano, Ciliberto and Ferrari 2012]. In this case, social judgement paralyzes Isabel, even with respect to individual and relational aspects. Taking a multi-process perspective, the therapist will help Isabel to come to terms with her being gay, to value the meaning attributed to it as a constitutive structure of her being. But a conversation about this cannot be separated from the consideration of the effects that being gay in a context that tends to be homophobic can have on the construction of the Self (see Box 10.2) to help her to combat internalized homophobia and increase positive gay identity. On the other hand, the loyalty she feels towards her parents leads her to not expose them to what she thinks could be painful by virtue of the prejudice about same-sex relationships. From this point of view, the therapist will help Isabel reflect on how much her parents and her sisters, in the name of their love for her, can support her instead. But in doing so, the therapist cannot forget Hannah, who is affirming her desire to realize their plans as a couple. So, the therapist will also invite Isabel to reflect on how much, for her sake, Hannah is willing to give her time, to wait for all the implications linked to the identity process and to the old (the family of origin) and new (the family of choice) relational involvements to be addressed and freed from the knots produced by the weight of social prejudices. Also, in this case, the therapist helps the client to rebuild herself as a person, to strengthen her relationships with others, and to cope with the exhaustion that being a member of a discriminated minority entails.

Box 10.2   Psychological effects of discrimination on the LGBT+ population

Self-invalidation

"Clinicians must be aware of the ubiquitous system of persecution of LGBT+ people and their families and consider the possible consequence that this generates ... Every LGBT+ person must deal with the devaluation acted in the family, school, work context – considered therefore natural and structural – that attacks the most intimate core of self-esteem and security. It is this internalized devaluation that prevents one from relating to and imagining oneself in ways, values and purposes that are as propositional and valid as the heterosexual individuals. This violence of invalidation, unconsciously assumed by the subject, reaches its goal: it becomes self-invalidation" [Rigliano *et al.* 2012, pp. 24–25].

Minority stress

Meyer's minority stress theory [2003] postulates that LGB individuals suffer several unique minority stressors in addition to the stressors normally experienced by heterosexual individuals because of their minority position. These unique minority stressors have a negative impact on the health of LGB individuals. The concept of social stress extends stress theory by suggesting that conditions in the social environment, and not only personal events, are sources of stress that affect the mental health of minorities. Individuals who belong to minorities may experience conditions such as conflicts, prejudice, discrimination, and stigma due to conflict with the social norms and structure set by the dominant culture for the entire society. According to Meyer, the main factors involved in the minority stress model are: 1) experiencing discrimination and victimization (prejudice event); 2) expectations of rejection and discrimination; 3) concealment of sexual orientation; and 4) internalized homophobia [Mongelli *et al.* 2019, p. 28].

Internalized homophobia

Internalized homophobia represents "the gay person's direction of negative social attitudes toward the self", and in its extreme forms, it can lead to the rejection of one's sexual orientation. Internalized homophobia is further characterized by an intrapsychic conflict between experiences of same-sex affection or desire and feeling a need to be heterosexual [Frost and Meyer 2009, p. 97]

Internalization of prejudices and psychotherapy

Prejudices are endemic in social communities, especially in periods of social change. Faced with new lifestyles, recognition of new rights, and legitimization of new needs emerging from the socio-cultural, demographic, legislative, and technological transformations that periodically occur in communities, common sense tends to anchor to the old knowledges, looking with suspicion and negativity at anything unusual. Whatever is unfamiliar and different is perceived as a threat to the social order and is rejected through discriminatory judgements and practices. So, LGBT+ people are considered sick, the use of assisted fertilization methods a shame, marital separation a fault, etc. All this occurs even though scientific research has amply demonstrated the contrary and the legislation of many countries has transformed the research results into institutional procedures and civil rights.

What is relevant from a therapeutic point of view, is that prejudices and stereotypes are often shared by people who belong to discriminated groups. The internalization of negative social judgements is often an obstacle to the effective mobilization of personal and emotional resources needed to cope with daily tasks, and it might trigger dysfunctional dynamics. When working with people belonging to groups subject to social prejudice, therapists must explore the extent to which the discomfort derives from choices made by people based on a shared social sentiment that, however, does not fit their psychological and material needs. The following are some examples: having the traditional nuclear family as a reference model when one is a member of a family with divorced or remarried parents; considering biological parenting as the only true form of parenting when one cannot have biological children; believing that relationships need constant presence when one is forced to live apart; thinking, in short, that the ideal way of being is what one is not, leads one to make choices that are dysfunctional and can create profound individual and family discomfort. Let's look at the following case.

Timothy is 18 years old and attends Classical Lyceum. One day, he unexpectedly attempts suicide. He is hospitalized, and during the hospitalization, his parents meet the psychologist, who collects the family history. Timothy's parents, Sandra and Andrew, have been divorced for 4 years because Sandra fell in love with a work colleague, Nolan, with whom she went to live. Following the separation of his parents, Timothy moved in with his mother and Nolan. The latter is in turn separated with 2 children, a son of 18 years and a girl of 13, who live with their mother and go to Nolan and Sandra's house periodically.

During the meeting, Timothy acts silly, laughs, and says he is well and there is no need to dramatize. He asks his parents to take him home. At a certain point, his father turns around, looks at him. and says: "Now stop being silly. The problem is serious. Let's figure out what to do". Timothy runs out of the room; when stopped by the nurse, he bursts into tears, admitting that he is not well. He says he does not know how to decide what to do in the future (choice of university), he feels empty, and he wants to die. He is paralyzed. His mother in turn bursts into tears, claiming that Timothy is sick because of the parents' divorce.

The psychologist notes that the father's restraining intervention had an impact on Timothy, and she thinks that the father can be a resource. As to the mother's explanation for Timothy's distress (the parents' divorce is the cause according to her), the psychologist observes that there are no elements to think that the divorce has grafted dysfunctional dynamics between Timothy and his parents: the father and mother have no conflicts; when the father intervened, the mother let it happen, thus authorizing the direct relationship between the father and son. The father takes responsibility for his role; there seems to be no triangulation or conflict of loyalties. Yet, the mother has the belief that she harmed her son with the divorce, and such a belief must be considered.

After a period of 15 days, the boy is discharged with a pharmacological prescription, with the advice to Timothy and his father to spend more time together, and with the recommendation to undertake family therapy. The parents agree with the psychologist, who had already met them to start the therapy. However, the psychologist specifies that she would like to see Timothy and all the adults who interact with him – therefore, his parents and Nolan, his mother's partner, because Timothy lives with his mother and him. They all accept the request. The psychologist notes that nobody opposes Nolan's presence at the family meetings, and therefore considers that there does not seem to be any role conflict between the different parental figures, who in fact can coexist in the same context. Obviously, there are other connections to look for.

Sandra, Nolan, Andrew, and Timothy go to the meeting as requested. Timothy is better, but not well. He still has the obsessive thoughts about what to do after high school. He goes more often to stay with his father, with whom he usually gets along well, but when he is anxious, he wants his father to call his mother. The explanation that Timothy wants to unite his parents is still not convincing the therapist, because although it is the most salient from a common sense perspective, there is no evidence consistent with that interpretation. The idea that Timothy wants to separate his mother from Nolan does not seem to have merit either. Why would Timothy want this after 4 years?

The therapist explores the relationships between the adult figures, especially between the father figures present in Timothy's daily life. Andrew affirms that he trusts Nolan, who in turn says that he loves Timothy like a son. The 2 men appear very confident in making these statements. Finally, Timothy is asked who he includes in his family, and he puts in everyone, even Nolan's children. For Timothy, the boundaries of his family are widened! The therapist wonders how the relationships within those boundaries are. Research on remarried families has long identified that there are 3 factors that above all contribute to the good functioning of remarried families and the well-being of the members [Visher, Visher and Pasley 2003]: the creation of a strong bond between the new couple; the development of a satisfactory relationship between the stepparents and children; and a mutual recognition of the different members of the extended family. The therapist reflects that of these 3 factors, the third one has been repeatedly observed as present in Timothy's family; in fact, no elements have emerged that would suggest a conflict between the 2 households (Sandra, Nolan, his children, and Timothy on one side; Andrew and Timothy on the other). On the contrary, there seems to be a healthy collaboration. The first 2 factors, however, need to be further explored, especially considering that Sandra persists in attributing the cause of Timothy's discomfort to her decision to divorce and move in with Nolan. Despite the validity of this research, it is frequently found that the members of remarried families have internalization of the negative judgement that common sense prejudicially assigns to divorce, but even more so to the formation of a new couple, both of which are considered reasons of distress for children. The therapist therefore decides to investigate the relational dynamics within the households.

It turns out that Nolan and Sandra practically lead separate lives, each with their own children. When Nolan's kids go to their house, Sandra and Timothy stay in one part of the house, and Nolan and his kids stay in another part. When Timothy goes to his father's house, Sandra stays alone because she fears that Timothy could be jealous of Nolan's children. The therapist connects this information with the fact that when Timothy is at his father's house he feels better, but when he has anxiety, he asks his father to call his mother, who in fact goes to them and is therefore no longer alone.

The therapist hypothesizes that because of Sandra's strong belief that divorce/remarriage has caused harm to her son, she has always tried to keep Timothy separated from Nolan in an ambiguous family ménage where relationships are both affirmed and denied. The therapist invites only Sandra and Nolan to the next meeting with the intention of talking about the relational organization of their domestic life. Nolan says he is unhappy and tired of the situation; he would like to change it, but Sandra does not want to because she fears for Timothy. She is convinced that Timothy wants her. He looks for her and calls her; therefore, she must reassure him that she is available despite everything.

The therapist explores the relationship between Sandra and Nolan, which seems to be solid in terms of their mutual feelings, but they fear that their love may harm others, and this belief organizes their family relationships. The therapists then decides to invite everyone to the next session, thinking that they need to be helped to find ways of mutual reassurance that instead of maintaining separate relationships, they can create more interdependence among the different relational contexts present in their extended family. She asks Nolan if he can reassure Timothy that when he goes to his father's house, his mother is not alone because she is with him and his children. And she asks Timothy to reassure his mother that he is fine with his father and he does not mind if she spends time with Nolan and his children. She asks Timothy if he can help his mother by spending time with Nolan's children so that she and Nolan can have time by themselves. She asks the father if Timothy can go to his place not on fixed days but depending on the situation that is created in the other household to give Nolan and Sandra the possibility of spending time with Nolan's children. He asks Nolan and Sandra if they can spend time with the 3 children so that Timothy's father can in turn have his time. At the end of the meeting, everyone is relieved. In the following months, the situation gradually improves. Timothy finally decides what university studies he will follow, and he and Nolan's children spend time together.

It is important for therapists to bear in mind the possibility that clients may internalize social prejudices or stereotypes and thus make decisions that end up not working within the new relational situation, creating individual and collective discomfort. But it is also important that psychotherapists first distance themselves from the prejudices that clients may have internalized. If the therapist in the above case had unknowingly shared the same prejudices as the clients, she would not have been able to conduct therapy as she did and would rather have confirmed the ideas they had. In this regard, the acquisition of awareness of one's own premises and the deconstruction of dominant "naturalized" beliefs, which we discussed in Chapters 5 and 6, are fundamental skills for psychotherapists to avoid colluding with their clients in confirming those ideas that lead to choices that produce discomfort

Adapting psychotherapeutic models to social transformations

In the chapters included in this fourth part of the book, we reflected on the sensitivity to context that therapists need to acquire to position themselves in the interweaving of individual, interpersonal, and social processes in which their intervention is embedded. We have defined the construct in various ways: knowing how to read the interdependence and co-evolution of the different relational contexts involved; building interdependent and co-ordinated networks; and conducting a multi-process analysis of distress and well-being. But there is another meaning that we would like to propose here. Context-sensitive therapists are also attentive to the socio-cultural-economic-institutional-technological transformations taking place in the context in which they practice and reflect on the technical, relational, and ethical adaptations that these transformations require with respect to their models. The radical changes we have witnessed in recent years have called for an honest and self-critical rethinking on the part of psychotherapists about their theoretical premises, their methodological principles, the concepts at the basis of their models of intervention, and their languages, to maintain a curious look at people's experiences and avoid placing them in predefined categories.

Reflections on language have proved to be fundamental in maintaining a position with clients that recognizes the subjectivity of the other and promotes a dialogue that is inclusive of different specificities. Think of the importance of not using sexist linguistic expressions when meeting with clients, to avoid taking a heterosexual orientation for granted. Questions such as "Are you currently in a romantic relationship?" is always preferable to "Do you have a boyfriend/girlfriend?"

Faced with the dynamics linked to divorce, couples' remarriage, inter-culturality, migration, inter-family solidarity, new forms of parenting, the spread of mediated communication, and the ageing of the population, family therapists have reflected on how much their models of intervention were still too tied to an idea of the traditional nuclear family and therefore inadequate to grasp the processes of families that differ in structure, foundation, and life circumstances. From this reflection, they developed new constructs suitable to capture the specificities of contemporary families.

In correspondence with empirical research that has documented the psychological and social well-being of children of same-sex couples, psychoanalysts have undertaken a critical revision of their models, critiquing the reification of the Oedipal scenario, and emphasizing how it represents an evolutionary model that describes the process through which boys and girls find their place within the family scene; a model therefore subjected to historical, geographical, and environmental variations of families.

On the other hand, as we have illustrated in the previous paragraphs, economic crises and migratory movements have led psychotherapists to historicize their models by integrating them with institutional, legal, and geopolitical references to be able to help people reconstruct identities that have been systematically trampled upon and thus to recover their ability to proactively face the challenges of their lives.

Today (Spring 2020), as we write, the entire Italian population, and other countries as well, are locked down as a measure of contrast to the pandemic produced by the spread of the Covid-19 virus; the quarantine has required the movement online of most activities, including psychotherapy. This is only the latest event that has urged therapists to reflect on what needs to be changed so that the setting of the encounter with the client remains, even at a distance, a setting of care – a personal, welcoming space suitable for mobilizing the relational resources that, as we have documented in this volume, constitute the driving force of change.

References

Afuape, T. [2016], *A 'Fifth Wave' systemic practice punctuating liberation: reflective practice and collective social action*, in I. McCarthy and G. Simon (eds.), *Systemic therapy as transformative practice*, Farnhill UK, Everything is Connected Press, pp.43–61.

Afuape, K., Bisimwa, N., Campbell, K., Jemmott, R., Jude, J., Nijabat, N., Olorunoje, M. and Simpson, S. [2022], *Black and proud: impact of intergenerational racism upon global majority family systems*, in Journal of Family Therapy, 44,1, pp. 5–19.

Afuape, T. and Kerry Oldham, S. (2022) *Beyond 'solidarity' with Black Lives Matter: drawing on liberation psychology and transformative justice to address institutional and community violence in young Black lives*, in Journal of Family Therapy, 44,1, pp. 20–43.

American Psychiatric Association [2000], *DSM-4-TR. Diagnostic and statistical manual of mental disorder. Text revision*, Arlington, VA, American Psychiatric Association.

American Psychiatric Association [2002], *DSM-5-TR Diagnostic and statistical manual of mental disorders. Text revision*, Arlington, VA, American Psychiatric Association.

Brondolo, E., Brady, N., Thompson, S., Tobin, J.N., Cassells, A., Sweeney, M., et al. [2008], *Perceived racism and negative affect: analyses of trait and state measures of affect in a community sample*, in Journal of Social and Clinical Psychology, 27, 2, pp. 150–173.

Brondolo, E., Brady ver Halen, N., Pencille, M., Beatty, D. and Contrada, R.J. [2009], *Coping with racism: a selective review of the literature and a theoretical and methodological critique*, in Journal of Behavioral Medicine, 32, pp. 64–88.

Chin, J., Hughes, G. , and Miller, A. [2022], *Examining our own relationships to racism as the foundation of decolonizing systemic practices.' No time like the present'*, in Journal of Family Therapy, 44, 1, pp. 76–90.

Conger, R.D., Conger, K.J. and Martin, M.J. [2010], *Socioeconomic status, family processes, and individual development*, in Journal of Marriage and Family, 72, pp. 685–704.

Cui, M., Donnellan, M.B. and Conger, R.D. [2007], *Reciprocal influences between parents' marital problems and adolescent internalizing and externalizing behavior*, in Developmental Psychology, 43, pp. 1544–1552.

Davolo, A. and Fruggeri, L. [2016], *A systemic-dialogical perspective for dealing with cultural differences in psychotherapy*, in I. McCarthy and G. Simon, (eds.), *Systemic therapy as transformative practice*, Farnhill UK, Everything is Connected Press, pp. 111–124.

Davolo, A. and Mancini, T. [2017], *L'intervento psicologico con i migranti*, Bologna, Il Mulino.

Frost, D.M. and Meyer, I.H. [2009]. *Internalized homophobia and relationship quality among lesbians, gay men, and bisexuals*, in Journal of Counseling Psychology, 56, 1, pp. 97–109.

Jones, E. [1993], *Family systems therapy*, ChiChester (UK), Wiley.

Jones, E. [1994], *Gender and poverty as context for depression*, in Human Systems. Special issue, 5, 3–4, pp. 169–183.

McCarthy [1994], *Poverty and social exclusion*, in Human Systems. Special issue, 5, 3–4, pp. 127–336.

McCarthy, I. (ed.) [1995], *Irish family studies: selected papers*, UCD, Family Studies Center.

McDowell, T., Libal, K. and Brown, A.L. [2012], *Human rights in the practice of family therapy: domestic violence, a case in point*, in Journal of Feminist Family Therapy, 24, 1, pp. 1–23.

Meyer, I.H. [2003], *Prejudice, social stress, and mental health in lesbian, gay, and bisexual populations: conceptual issues and research evidence*, in Psychol Bull, 129, pp. 674–697.

Mongelli, F., Perrone, D., Balducci, J., Sacchetti, A., Ferrari, S., Mattei, G. and Galeazzi, G.M. [2019], *Minority stress and mental health among LGBT populations: an update on the evidence*, in Minerva Psichiatrica, 60, 1, pp. 27–50.

Nelson, J.A., O'brien, M., Blankson, A.N., Calkins, S.D. and Keane, S.P. [2009], *Family stress and parental responses to children's negative emotions: tests of the spillover, crossover, and compensatory hypotheses*, in Journal of Family Psychology, 23, pp. 671–679.

Nievar, M.A. and Luster, T. [2006], *Developmental processes in African American families: an application of McLoyd's theoretical model*, in Journal of Marriage and Family, 68, pp. 320–331.

Pakman, M. [1997], *La micro-politica delle classi sociali nella vita familiare*, in Connessioni, 2, pp. 24–33.

Rigliano, P., Ciliberto, J. and Ferrari, F. [2012], *Curare i gay? Oltre l'ideologia riparativa dell'omosessualità*, Milano, Raffaello Cortina.

Sironi, F. [2007], *Psychopathologie des violences collectives. Essai de psychologie géopolitique clinique*, Paris, Odil Jacob.

Todd, N. and Wade, A. [2003], *Coming to terms with violence and resistance: from a language of effects to a language of responses*, in T. Strong and D. Pare (eds.), *Furthering talk: advances in the discursive therapies*, New York, Kluwer Academic Plenum, pp. 145–161.

Visher, E.B., Visher, J.S. and Pasley, K. [2003], *Remarriage families and stepparenting*, in F. Walsh (ed.), *Normal family processes (3rd edition)*, The Guilford Press, New York, pp. 153–175.

Walters, M. [1990], *A feminist perspective in family therapy*, in R.J. Perelberg and A.C. Miller (eds.) *Gender and power in families*, London, Routledge, pp. 13–33.

Williams, D.R. and Mohammed, S.A. [2009], *Discrimination and racial disparities in health: evidence and needed research*, in Journal of Behavioral Medicine, 32, pp. 20–47.

Concluding remarks. Beyond psychotherapy

Studies that have empirically verified the specific and non-specific factors that most influence the success of psychotherapies have documented those characteristics of therapists that positively influence treatment outcomes. As we reported in the Introduction, the most effective therapists are those who are able to create a good alliance with their clients; have good interpersonal skills; are flexible, open, respectful, and interested in their clients; do not impose their beliefs on clients, but listen to what their clients bring to therapy; are self-confident, but able to question themselves; monitor their clients' change within a collaborative dialogue; are aware of their own internal processes and emotions, and do not let these unconsciously interfere with the therapeutic process; and are able to use them deliberately for clinical purposes [Ackerman and Hilsenroth 2003; Wampold and Carlson 2011; Wampold 2015; Norcross and Lambert 2018]. These ways of being and acting are relational and epistemological postures that cut across models; in fact, they concern the *how*, not the what, of psychotherapists' work. They evoke second-level abilities that pertain to the construction and monitoring of the therapeutic process.

Defining certain therapeutic competencies as transmodel does not mean that they are entrusted to the discretion of the individual therapist. On the contrary, they can and must be the object of teaching and learning. The therapeutic competencies, which we have illustrated in this volume, are skills that support the postures listed above, we could even say that they constitute their methodological and operationalised expressions. In fact, the ability to build with clients a symbolic shared dialogic space, also possibly resorting to technical devices (cf. Chapters 1 and 2), allows monitoring their change collectively. The creation of a good alliance is a process that requires knowledge of the factors that contribute to its construction and of the tools that allow monitoring its development (cf. Chapter 3). The ability to read the joint action, the dance to which therapist and patient give shape during their encounters, provides the methodological criteria to decide when and whether it is appropriate to use for clinical purposes one's own emotions or to make an intervention that is unorthodox with respect to one's own model (cf. Chapter 4). The relational competency that allows acknowledging the development of the therapeutic process and detecting what the therapist and client build together is a necessary condition for questioning one's own work. Awareness of one's own premises and the epistemological exercises illustrated in the third part of the book are the essential tools to become aware of one's own internal processes and prevent them from unconsciously interfering with the therapeutic process. Curiosity, decentring, and distinguishing reasons from solutions are methodological paths that favour being flexible, open, respectful, and interested in clients, without imposing one's own beliefs on them, but staying tuned to what they tell.

Psychotherapy is an activity that involves different levels of intrapersonal, interpersonal, social, cultural, and institutional processes. For this reason, to the dialogical, relational, and reflexive skills of therapists we have added the acknowledgement of the context, that is the ability to build networks and to include the interpersonal and social contexts in which clients live and in which therapy takes place and develops. It is a competency that allows therapists to historicize the models adopted to be able to grasp the influence of social, political, cultural, and economic processes on the well-being/discomfort of individuals, to avoid psychologising or personalising distress and suffering that originate at the macro-societal level.

We have described and exemplified the above psychotherapeutic competencies in such a way as to grasp their core methodological aspects, and as such, they can be the object of teaching and learning. Relational and epistemological competency, and acknowledgement of the context, can be considered trans-model competencies, useful when the technique does not help to get out of impasse situations. Those are the moments when therapists should assume a self-reflective position to analyse the relationship with the patient, to reflect on one's own premises, to change one's perspective, to adopt a co-evolutionary and multi-processual view, and to reintroduce flexibility and generativity in the therapeutic process.

The competencies described in this book, being related to the interpersonal and social construction processes that constitute the plot of an intervention, can be a valid reference also for other professionals working in social, educational, and health services.

In the medical field, for example, the model of "patient-centred medicine" has documented the importance of communication and relationship in the process of health treatment [Nova, Vegni and Moja 2005], and in this regard, physicians are the first to request training courses that include these issues [Lamiani et al. 2011]. If it is fundamental that a doctor makes a correct diagnosis to identify the correct treatment, it is equally important how the diagnosis is communicated to the patient. Developing relational competency for medical doctors means overcoming communication based on rigid and predefined protocols, to enhance instead the understanding of the interaction with that patient and to evaluate situation by situation the most appropriate communication modalities. For example, the relational competency of paediatricians allow them, during a diagnosis of disability, to explore the fears and worries of the parents to evaluate how these can interfere with the collaboration necessary for the continuation of the diagnostic and therapeutic-rehabilitation process. The alliance between doctor and patient, which is so important for the success of the treatment, has characteristics that are not dissimilar to the alliance between client and psychotherapist. It is indeed important for patients to feel welcomed in their fears and doubts, to trust that the doctor will solve their problems, to feel that the doctor cares about them. In this sense, knowing how to decentre would also help the construction of the alliance, since the doctor would be prepared, by trying to take the patient's perspective, to grasp the fragility and insecurity that a person often feels in the face of illness. Moreover, some health professionals, such as paediatricians and midwives, meet patients from different family forms and are urged to be self-reflective to avoid relating to them with prejudice and discriminatory attitudes. For example, community paediatricians, to whom heterosexual couples who have resorted to heterologous fertilisation entrust their anxieties and dilemmas (should they or should they not tell their child? if yes, how?), are unable to provide the help they require without first reflecting on how they evaluate this choice. Midwifes may encounter among the women and couples they assist before, during, and after childbirth, persons that are exposed to social prejudices, such as lesbian couples, or people confined to the area of social exclusion, such as women with psychiatric problems or addictions; for these professionals, it is necessary to reflect on their own premises to avoid unconscious differences in treatment and improper judgements. Especially when working with clients belonging to different cultures, they need to take a curious stance towards non-western understanding of illness and disability.

Family diversity and multiculturalism have also urged educators and teachers to reflect on what idea of the family guides their daily work and to focus on the prejudices and social stereotypes still present in the practices, languages, and documents through which the educational services carry out their mission [Everri *et al.* 2021]. In education, acknowledging the context to which children and adolescents belong is also important. The concepts of "interdependence" and "co-evolution" are particularly significant conceptual tools, given that the context of belonging has a central function in the development of children. Developing this competency allows, in fact, to organise one's intervention not simply based on what one thinks useful and evolving for the child but based on what one thinks useful and evolving for the child as a member of a family system. It is precisely those who work in the educational field who cannot ignore the teaching of Bronfenbrenner [1979], who reminds us that a dyad is evolutionary only insofar as it has positive repercussions in other relational contexts connected to it. The implementation of this skill recalls relational competency. It is the educators' duty to communicate to parents any problems observed about their child, but it is essential that they pay attention to how they do so, to avoid the parents feeling judged incompetent, and in general, it is important that they take care in building an alliance with the parents to create a positive relational context in which even the most thorny issues can be addressed in a collaborative and evolutionary way. Finally, empirical studies document how the relational aspect also concerns learning processes: quality teaching is achieved when teachers treat learning as a social and communicative process [Rojas-Drummond and Mercer 2003; Molinari and Mameli 2013].

Professionals working in social services often need to develop epistemological competency. Social workers are particularly involved with people who live on the margins of society, people about whom the collective judgement is often merciless, people who do not think they can cope, and people who suffer due to social exclusion. The epistemological exercises described in the third part of this volume would greatly help social workers to introduce hope into their interventions. In this sense, the deconstruction of socially established and dominant ideas is not only required of psychologists and psychotherapists. The importance of going beyond the behaviours, i.e., the dysfunctional solutions or strategies that people adopt, in order to reach people's deep reasons and needs is a fundamental methodological principle for those who work in the area of social marginalization, since it is precisely the most socially fragile people who resort to shortcuts or dysfunctional solutions, which in turn leaves their needs unsatisfied and places them in useless and sometimes degrading welfare circuits [Fruggeri and Matteini 1994; McCarthy 2001].

Finally, the ability to conceive of oneself as within a network, as we discussed in Chapter 9, is a competency that concerns all professionals, who, although starting within different fields, find themselves collaborating and coordinating for the same case.

Each profession has, of course, its own specific techniques and procedures, but educational, social, and health interventions also take place within an interweaving of processes that connect personal aspects to inter-individual ones, and both to socio-economic-political-institutional ones. From this point of view, knowing how to promote and analyse the relationship with the client, knowing how to change perspective when interventions seem to reach a blind spot, valuing the other's point of view by practicing decentring, considering people's life contexts and the way they affect their system of meanings and relationships, and knowing how to conduct a multi-process analysis of the situations in which one intervenes, are skills that support any intervention carried out within the helping professions.

Bibliography

Ackerman, S.J. and Hilsenroth, M.J. [2003], *A review of therapist characteristics and techniques positively impacting the therapeutic alliance*, in Clinical Psychology Review, 23, 1, pp. 1–33.

Bronfenbrenner, U. [1979], *The ecology of human development*, Cambridge MA, Harvard University Press.

Everri, M., Mancini, T., O'Brian, V. and Fruggeri, L. [2021], Cultivating *practices of inclusion towards same-sex families in Italy: a comparison among educators, social workers, and healthcare professionals*, in Journal of Community & Applied Social Psychology, 31, pp. 659–672.

Fruggeri, L. and Matteini, M. [1994], *Poverty and social services*, in Human Systems, 5, 3-4, pp. 319–336.

Lamiani, G., Meyer, E.C., Leone, D., Vegni, E., Browning, D.M., Rider, E.A., Truog, R.D. and Moja, E.A. [2011], *Cross-cultural adaptation of an innovative approach to learning about difficult conversations in healthcare*, in Medical Teacher, 33, 2, pp. e57–e64.

McCarthy, I. [2001], *Fifth Province re-versings:1 the social construction of women lone parents' inequality and poverty*, in Journal of Family Therapy, 23, pp. 253–277.

Molinari, L. and Mameli, C. [2013], *Process quality of classroom discourse: pupil participation and learning opportunities*, in International Journal of Educational Research, 62, pp. 249–258.

Norcross, J.C. and Lambert, M.J. [2018], *Psychotherapy relationships that work III*, in Psychotherapy, 55, 4, pp. 303–315.

Nova, C., Vegni, E. and Moja, E.A. [2005], *The physician–patient–parent communication: a qualitative perspective on the child's contribution*, in Patient Education and Counseling, 58, 3, pp. 327–333.

Rojas-Drummond, S. and Mercer, N. [2003], *Scaffolding the development of effective collaboration and learning*, in International Journal of Educational Research, 39, 1-2, pp. 99–111.

Wampold, B.E. [2015], *How important are the common factors in psychotherapy? An update*, in World Psychiatry, 14, 3, pp. 270–277.

Wampold, B.E. and Carlson, J. [2011], *Qualities and actions of effective therapists*, Washington DC, American Psychological Association.

Index

Page numbers followed by "n" indicate notes.

assessment 5, 20–21, 23, 53, 60; parenting 52, 162, 163

belief 6, 38, 39, 99–100, 106, 181; awareness of 11, 107, 137, 116–117, 177; deconstructing 113, 116–117, 119; naturalized beliefs 11, 117, 137, 177; organizing family relationships 175, 176; in therapeutic interventions 37, 39–42, 51
bona fide treatment 5, 12n2

care 119, 148, 161, 167, 183; setting of 23, 178; system of 152, 157–158; in therapeutic alliance 58, 64
change 2, 5, 23–25, 28, 85; point of view 11, 97–98, 123, 127; process of 62, 107, 141; social change 167–168, 174, 177; support change 21, 41, 46–47, 125, 164
circularity 28, 41–42, 161
class *see* social class
co-evolution 12, 26–27, 141, 145, 183; co-evolution of systems 143; co-evolutionary perspective 143, 150, 154, 182; co-evolutionary practice 26; co-evolutionary process 27, 42, 148
common factors 2, 5, 10, 61
common sense 11, 24, 100–101, 128, 137
complementarity 113–114, 116, 125n1, 159
complex thinking 99, 137, 161; fostering of 120, 123
connection 175; among professionals 157; with client's story 25, 129; of descriptions 48; of events 42, 106; generation of new connections 43; of interventions 156; of meanings 86, of opposites 113, 116, 137; of pieces of information 24, 42

construction/co-construction/social construction 1, 10; of alliance 9, 11, 58, 183; analysis/monitoring of co-construction process 92, 181; individual/joint construction 75–81; of meanings, identities, relationships, realities 10–11, 57, 66, 75, 105, 117; of psychopathology 100; of a shared symbolic space/transformative context 9, 23–26, 51, 64, 72, 161; of therapeutic dialogue 36–53; of the therapeutic process 86–88
construction of the self 172
constructionism 1, 20, 33, 51, 161
contemporary families *see* families
context 1, 19, 23, 127–128, 141; acknowledging the 11, 141–145, 164, 166, 170, 177; interactive 24, 82–83, 85, 88; of interpersonal relationship 142–143, 145, 152, 161, 163–164, 167; social 107, 167–168; in therapeutic interventions 20, 39–40, 41, 43, 46, **47**, 48–49; transformative 9, 10, 53, 58, 86
conversation 20, 26, 168; analysis of 83; conducting a 28; development of 23–24, 31, 36, 41, 47; on the identities 64, 108–109
coordination 1; of professionals 153, 157, 161
culture 31, 107, 117; dominant 113, 135, 173; minority 32, 70, 183
curiosity 21, 99, 127–128, 131, 137

decentring 9, 44, 128, 129, 134, 137
decolonizing practice 32, 109, 168
diagnosis 9, 19, 20–21, 121, 182
dialogism 26–27, 154

dialogue 25, 27, 82, 153–154, 170, 177; on the identities 109; internal 26, 28, 78, 81, 89; transformative 10, 37, 47, 51, 53

differences/information of difference 21, 24, 42, 53, 123, 128, 163; *see also* Social differences

discrimination 31–32, 167, 168, 170, 173

divergent thinking 21, 123–125

dominant beliefs, class, culture, discourse, values, and norms 113, 116–117, 166, 173, 177, 184; clients' dominant story 27, 46; *see also* Common sense; and Self-reflexivity

double vision 89, 92

emotional connection 58, 61–62, 65–67, 82

emotions 75, 129, 134, 161, 181; of the therapist 25, 66, 103, 105–106, 117

engagement 41, 61–62, 70–72

epistemology 98–99, 113

ethnicity 32, 64, 107–108

evidence based practice 7

exploration 41, 87, 103, 110, 134

families: discourse 82; functioning 114, 167; interactions 142, 145, 163; types of 117, 174, 178, 183

feedback 24, 28, 36, 43, 88, 107

feelings: client's 25, 59, 64, 65, 91, 142; questions about 37, 39, 44; therapists' 66, 79, 97, 105

gender 12, 40, 64, 107–110, 117, 167

hypothesis 23–25, 27, 28, 84, 97, 98

hypothesising 25, 36, 99

identities 81, 82–83, 85, 121, 143; disclosure of 64, 108–109

impasse 97, 103, 105, 114, 182

individual construction *see* construction

information: 9, 10, 19, 21, 23, 25; circularity 154, 161, 164; collecting 36, 38, 39, 40, 45, 52

inner dialogue *see* dialogue

interdependence 12, 24–25, 143, 152–154, 166, 183

intersubjectivity 10

irreverence 102

joint construction *see* construction

knowledge 98–100; professional 11, 19, 78, 116–117; *see also* common sense

language 100, 109, 177

loyalty conflict 142

manualisation 3, 9, 60

map 8, 21, 51, 105

meanings 81, 88, 131, 150, 157, 166; attribution of 24, 77–78, 172; meaning making process 25, 57–58, 65, 97, 129, 164; system of 141, 143

metaphorical techniques 51, 52

minorities 31, 32, 172, 173

multiple descriptions 120, 137

multi-process analysis 166, 170, 172, 177

narrative 36, 46–51, 105, 127–128

naturalized beliefs *see* beliefs

network 27, 100, 154–155, 161, 184; of relationship 9, 19, 24, 141–142, 148, 152; of therapist/ professional 12, 19, 117, 152–153, 157, 182

observational tool 51–52, 60

opposites *see* connection of opposites

oppression 31, 109, 134, 167–168

outcome 59, 60, 76, 121, 123, 181; positive 58, 66, 81, 143, 157, 161; psychotherapy 2–9, 67, 137

pattern 22, 46, 78, 125, 127, 155; which connects 41, 113; family 9, 19, 52; of interaction 42, 49, 105

position/positioning 42, 82, 85, 104, 128, 145; social 64, 78, 100, 107, 137; therapist's 28, 31, 66, 117, 137, 150

power 12, 31–32, 64, 81, 107–109, 166

poverty 12, 31, 132, 167

prejudices 25, 78–79, 107, 117, 137; social 100, 166, 170–174, 177, 183; therapist's 11, 25, 131

premises 1, 11, 19, 36, 122, 167; client's 6, 127–128; therapist's 9, 25, 78, 137, 177, 182–183

psychopathology 20, 22, 24, 100, 122, 127

racism/race/racial 32, 64, 108–109, 117, 168–170

reasons/goals 131, 134, 137

recursivity 78, 81, 98, 136

reflexivity 9–11, 36, 51, 91, 127, 136; *see also* Self-reflexivity

resources: of the community 46, 53;
    mobilizing resources of clients 10, 21,
    41, 52, 92, 105; of the network of
    professionals 153, 161; personal
    resources 174; valuing resources 12,
    122–124, 153, 167–168
responsibility 44, 50, 154, 162, 168, 170;
    parental 123, 175; therapist 97, 86, 91
rights 118, 119, 170, 174

safety 59, 61–64
second order: concept 128; position 9, 85;
    competency 82
self 37, 106–107, 114, 121–122, 163–164,
    172–173; Self-awareness 32, 78, 99, 103,
    105; *see also* beliefs; self-disclosure 108;
    self-healing 5; self -observation 106; self-
    referential 25, 136; self-reflexivity 11,
    99–101, 107–110, 119, 136, 182–183;
    self-validating/self-invalidation 99, 173
sexual orientation 65, 107, 110, 171,
    173, 177
skills: therapists' skills 6–11, 27, 51, 78, 177,
    181–183; clients' skills 10
shared sense of purpose 61–62, 67, 69–70
social actor 11, 99–100, 123
social class 40, 100, 107, 108
social construction *see* construction
social differences 12, 31, 64, 107–109,
    137n1, 167
social representations 100, 116–117, 166

social status 31, 64, 81, 137, 167
specific factors 2–7, 181
strategizing 28, 78
symptom 9, 19–20, 24, 47–50, 52, 83;
    symptoms and social status 167–169
System for Observing Family Therapy
    Alliances (SOFTA) *see* therapeutic
    alliance

therapeutic alliance 10, 57–60, 108, 183; as
    common factor 6–9; dimensions of 62,
    64–71; promoting the 82, 91; split
    alliance 59–60; System for Observing
    Family Therapy Alliances (SOFTA)
    60–62, 66–67, 72n1
therapeutic plan 156–160, 163
training 6, 11, 78, 105–107, 109, 182
trauma 169
triadic: triadic coevolution *see* co-evolution;
    triadic hypothesis 24; triadic interaction/
    interactional context 24, 30, 52,
    142–143, 162–16; Triadic Interaction
    Analytical Procedures (TIAP) 52, 162,
    164; triadic perspective 24, 148

unintended consequences 76–77, 87

validity 2–3
violence 128–129, 142, 173; collective
    violence 168–169; institutional violence
    134; victims of violence 46, 128